RENAL DIET COOKBOOK

Text Copyright ©

All rights reserved. No part of this guide may be reproduced in any form without permission in writing from the publisher except in the case of brief quotations embodied in critical articles or reviews.

Legal & Disclaimer

The information contained in this book and its contents is not designed to replace or take the place of any form of medical or professional advice; and is not meant to replace the need for independent medical, financial, legal or other professional advice or services, as may be required. The content and information in this book has been provided for educational and entertainment purposes only.

The content and information contained in this book has been compiled from sources deemed reliable, and it is accurate to the best of the Author's knowledge, information and belief. However, the Author cannot guarantee its accuracy and validity and cannot be held liable for any errors and/or omissions. Further, changes are periodically made to this book as and when needed. Where appropriate and/or necessary, you must consult a professional (including but not limited to your doctor, attorney, financial advisor or such other professional advisor) before using any of the suggested remedies, techniques, or information in this book.

Upon using the contents and information contained in this book, you agree to hold harmless the Author from and against any damages, costs, and expenses, including any legal fees potentially resulting from the application of any of the information provided by this book. This disclaimer applies to any loss, damages or injury caused by the use and application, whether directly or indirectly, of any advice or information presented, whether for breach of contract, tort, negligence, personal injury, criminal intent, or under any other cause of action.

You agree to accept all risks of using the information presented inside this book.

You agree that by continuing to read this book, where appropriate and/or necessary, you shall consult a professional (including but not limited to your doctor, attorney, or financial advisor or such other advisor as needed) before using any of the suggested remedies, techniques, or information in this book.

Table of contents

Chapter 1: THE RENAL DIET 6
  What is Renal Diet? 6
  What the ingredients are and what they do in a renal diet lifestyle 7
  Phosphorus and How It Relates to Kidneys Disease 11
  Phosphorus in Food: How to Lower Phosphorus Levels Through Renal Diet ... 12
  Some Strategies/Tips on How to Behave During a Renal Diet 22
  Different stages of kidney disease. A little explanation 26

Chapter 2: THE RECIPES Breakfast Recipes 30
  1. Egg White and Pepper Omelet 31
  2. Blueberry Smoothie Bowl 32
  3. Turkey Breakfast Sausage 33
  4. Italian Apple Fritters 34
  5. Tofu and Mushroom Scramble 35
  6. Sunny Pineapple Breakfast Smoothie 36
  7. Puff Oven Pancakes 37
  8. Savory Muffins with Protein 38
  9. European Pancakes 40
  10. Puffy French Toast 41
  11. Vegetable Rice Casserole 42
  12. Egg Fried Rice 44
  13. Mushroom Rice Noodles 46
  14. Mixed Vegetable Barley 48
  15. Spicy Sesame Tofu 50

Lunch Recipes 52
  16. Creamy Chicken with Cider 53

17.	Easy and Fast Mac-n-Cheese	54
18.	Exotic Palabok	55
19.	Vegetarian Gobi Curry	57
20.	Marinated Shrimp and Pasta	59
21.	Steak and Onion Sandwich	61
25.	Zucchini Noodles With Spring Vegetables	67
26.	Stir-Fried Vegetables	69
27.	Lime Asparagus Spaghetti	71
28.	Garden Crustless Quiche	73
29.	Lentil Veggie Burgers	75
30.	Baked Cauliflower Rice Cakes	77

Snacks Recipes 79

31.	Cinnamon Apple Chips	80
32.	Savory Collard Chips	81
33.	Roasted Red Pepper Hummus	83
34.	Thai-Style Eggplant Dip	85
35.	Collard Salad Rolls with Peanut Dipping Sauce	87
36.	Roasted Mint Carrots	89
37.	Roasted Root Vegetables	91
38.	Vegetable Couscous	93
39.	Garlic Cauliflower Rice	95
40.	Celery and Arugula Salad	97
41.	Cucumber and Radish Salad	99
42.	Spinach Salad with Orange Vinaigrette	100
43.	Mixed Green Leaf and Citrus Salad	101
44.	Roasted Beet Salad	103
45.	Pear and Watercress Salad	105

Dinner Recipes 107
1. Vegetable Lover's Chicken Soup 107
46. Creamy Pumpkin Soup 109
47. Broccoli, Arugula and Avocado Cream Soup 111
48. Salad Greens with Roasted Beets 112
49. Nutty and Fruity Garden Salad 113
50. Roasted Salmon Garden Salad 114
51. Rosemary Grilled Chicken 115
52. Creamy Egg Scramble on Cauliflower Pilaf 116
53. Roasted Veggies Mediterranean Style 117
54. Fruity Garden Lettuce Salad 118
55. Red Coleslaw with Apple 119
56. Roasted Cauliflower with Mixed Greens Salad 121
57. Bulgur and Broccoli Salad 123
58. Marinated Shrimp and Pasta 125
59. Steak and Onion Sandwich 127

Chapter 1: THE RENAL DIET

What is Renal Diet?

The renal diet is a dietary regimen designed to bring relief to patients with slow or damaged renal functions and chronic kidney diseases. As we have already mentioned at the end of Chapter one, there is no a single uniformed type of renal diet—this is the case because requirements of renal diet as well as restrictions, need to match the needs of the patient and be based on what doctor prescribed for the patient's overall health.

However, all forms of renal diet have one thing in common, which is to improve your renal functions, bring some relief to your kidneys, as well as prevent kidneys disease at patients with numerous risk factors, altogether improving your overall health and well-being. The grocery list we have provided should help you get ahold of which groceries you should introduce to your diet and which groups of food should be avoided in order to improve your kidneys' performance, so you can start from shopping for your new lifestyle.

You don't need to shop for many different types of groceries all at once as it is always better to use fresh produce, although frozen food also makes a good alternative when fresh fruit and vegetables are not available.

Remember to treat canned goods as suggested and recommended in the previous chapter and drain excess liquid from the canned food.

As far as the renal diet we are recommending in our guide, this form of kidney-friendly dietary regimen offers a solution in form of low-sodium and low-potassium meals and groceries, which is why we are also offering simple and easy renal diet recipes in our guide. By following a dietary plan compiled for all stages of renal system failure unless the doctor recommends a different treatment by allowing or expelling some of the groceries, we have listed in our ultimate grocery list for renal patients.

Before we get to the cooking and changing your lifestyle from the very core with the idea of improving your health, we want you to get familiar with renal diet basics and find out exactly what his diet is based on while you already know what is the very core solution found in the renal diet—helping you improve your kidney's health by lowering sodium and potassium intake.

The best way of getting familiar with the renal diet and basics of this dietary regimen is to take a look at the most commonly asked questions that extend the answer to a question. What is the renal diet?

What the ingredients are and what they do in a renal diet lifestyle

These are some of the most commonly asked questions that should clarify many of your doubts on what renal diet actually represents and stands for.

What is the renal diet based on?

The renal diet is a dietary regimen that restricts food groups that may bring harm to an already damaged renal system and kidneys. The main goal of the diet is to help patients who had already been diagnosed with a form of kidneys disease to live a healthier lifestyle, enabling them to manually regulate the presence of sodium, potassium, water, and waste that should be otherwise regulated by healthy kidneys and normal renal function. The renal diet is based on the introduction of foods that are low in sodium and potassium.

How much protein do I need for normal functions?

Protein requirements and needs may be different from patient to patient, but when talking in general, meat portions should be lowered to minimal consumption, while you may seek other sources of protein in alternative food options besides meat products such as beef and chicken. Protein is being processed by kidneys and since you are having issues with your renal functions, you need to lower your protein intake. Still, protein consumption should be kept at satisfying levels so your body would be able to function properly. Approximately, in case you are not a dialysis patient, the average protein intake should be anywhere between 0.8 grams of protein per kilogram of your body weight daily. In case you are a dialysis patient, the average intake of protein per day should be between 1 and 1.3 grams of protein per kilogram of your body weight. In case you have more kilograms than you are supposed to, it is recommended to lose weight in a healthy way with physical activity and a healthy diet regimen. Protein helps our body heal in a way, as the presence of protein in our blood called albumin regulates growth as well as repair of damaged tissue, which is why protein is important.

Can I use meat substitutes for protein sources?

Patients with kidney disease that dislike or don't consume meat out of different reasons may find a valuable dose of daily protein intake through several alternatives. Even though low protein consumption is recommended when on a renal diet, you need to make sure that you are not neglecting the need your body has for protein. That is how renal patients that avoid eating meat need to find ways of taking protein through a daily diet in recommended doses. For instance, instead of meat and in case you can't eat even small portions of meat, you can turn to an animal-based protein found in cheese and eggs. Since only low-sodium and low-potassium cheese is allowed, make sure to find suitable alternatives in case you want to include cheese in your diet. Additionally, you need to talk to your doctor about the number of eggs and milk you are allowed to have on a daily and weekly basis. Moreover, you can use egg substitutes and protein shakes mixed with fruit that is suitable for your condition and your diet regimen.

Why is alcohol on the DON'T list in the renal diet?

Alcohol like wine and beer might be consumed in a moderate manner if allowed by your doctor, however, general recommendations regarding alcohol when it comes to renal diet and the well-being of your renal functions, is to avoid alcohol at all costs. Alcohol may increase your blood pressure help you gain weight and increase the levels of blood sugar in your body. Additionally, alcohol introduces more toxic waste to your body for your kidneys to work against, which may bring more damage to your kidneys while also potentially damaging the liver and pancreas. On top of these risks when consuming alcohol, one of the main reasons why alcohol should be out of your range is due to the fact that alcohol shouldn't be mixed with medications that you are taking for your kidneys condition.

As for another important reason why alcoholic beverages should be avoided, is the fact that some alcohol drinks contain higher doses of potassium. For instance, red wine and beer have high concentrations of potassium, while spirits actually contain almost none. In case your doctor allows an occasional glass of wine, you should be fine, but try to avoid drinking alcohol.

Should I lower my liquid intake on a renal diet?

The renal diet recommends the reduction of liquid as one of the effective ways to help your kidneys and improve your renal function since damaged kidneys are struggling with removing excess water from your organism when liquid consumption is increased and above normal. However, only reduce your liquid intake if your doctor prescribes it as an unnecessary liquid reduction may cause more problems to your body and health. When it comes to beverages rather than water, avoid sugar-packed drinks and sodas.

What is low and what is considered high potassium in food?

Potassium levels vary from one food product to another, while some store-bought groceries with nutrition labels won't even list potassium—that does not mean that the food product necessarily contains no potassium, it only means that the manufacturer didn't consider that listing this mineral is essential. You can always do research on potassium levels on almost any food you are buying and consuming low levels of potassium is considered to be around 40 mg, while very high potassium levels are considered to be above 500 mg per serving, representing a concentration of 14% per portion.

Unless your doctor advises otherwise, you should lower your potassium intake to minimum levels for best results with the renal diet. However, you should remember that potassium is one of the essential minerals that your body needs, which is why you shouldn't completely neglect the consumption of potassium through food.

Should I take vitamins and herbal supplements while on the renal diet?

People with chronic kidneys disease may lack some essential vitamins that are categorized as water-soluble, while kidney patients that have dialysis treatment may lack these vitamins, such as groups of B vitamin. Other vitamins may lack as well regardless of diversity in your diet and despite the fact that you are eating enough healthy food that should provide your body with all the nutrients it needs for proper functioning. However, we do not recommend taking any supplements, herbal, or in the form of vitamin pills when on the renal diet unless, of course, prescribed by your doctor. Your doctor may accurately prescribe additional doses of vitamins in the form of supplements based on your blood test results and deeper knowledge on your health condition and the state of your disease. Do not take any supplements on your own and without consulting your doctor.

What can I do about my low appetite?

Low appetite and the inability to consume food on a regular basis is a common side-effect for patients that have problems with kidneys. This is the case because your kidneys are struggling to eject all the waste build up in your body. This state may cause loss of appetite in the long run, which is not good for your body. When you are not introducing nutrients to your organism, your body needs to find another source of nutrients in your body, drawing build up nutrients from reserves and first "eating out" fat reserves in your body then getting to your muscles.

You need to eat in order to prevent muscle loss and further damage to your health, however, eating with poor appetite may seem like a mission impossible. There are several things you can do in order to improve and boost your appetite even through hard times:

✓ Try setting up an eating schedule for yourself, and eat smaller portions of food that are packed with calories so that you can have as much energy and nutrients even though smaller portions of food when your appetite is lower. Try not to miss out on any scheduled meal that you have set up for yourself Fresh air and physical activity such as swimming, cycling, or even taking a walk may wake up your appetite and improve it.

✓ When on low appetite, try snacking on healthy snacks and eat more frequently in smaller portions.

✓ Make sure that your meals, even though small, have enough proteins and calories so you would prevent muscle loss and have the needed energy.

✓ Eating your favorite food may work benevolently on improving your appetite. Make sure that the food you like eating is low on potassium and sodium.

✓ Soups with added meat such as ground beef or chicken may be a great choice for you when you are having problems with eating as you will be able to introduce your body to essential nutrients through a light meal that you might be able to eat more easily than it would be the case with solid food.

✓ Add eggs and low-sodium cheese to salads when on low appetite to make sure that you are getting the nutrients you need even in case of poor appetite.

Can I Eat Whole Grains and Nuts on the Renal Diet?

The renal diet advises caution when it comes to the consumption of whole grains and nuts as these food groups have high concentrations of potassium. During checkups on your potassium levels as tested by your doctor, make sure to ask your physician whether you are allowed to eat whole grains and nuts. Patients who had just had a successful kidney transplant are recommended to have whole grains, nuts, and seeds, increased protein consumption in order to encourage tissue repair, as well as beans and lentils that are normally not the first food groups recommended in the renal diet.

Does the Renal Diet Work on Slowing Down the Progression of Chronic Kidneys Disease?

Even in case you are at the third stage of chronic kidneys disease, renal diet can help you improve your health as this diet is designed to improve the overall function of the renal system and kidneys, preventing further damage to your vital organs. However, the renal diet may not be as effective in case your lifestyle is not complementing the effects of a healthy diet that the renal dietary program represents. To get the most out of the renal diet, you also need to improve your lifestyle.

Besides eating healthy food as suggested in our grocery lists, you also need to introduce some physical activities to your everyday routine. As mentioned earlier in the book, you don't need to hire a personal trainer and sign up for a membership at your local gym. It would be enough to jog, walk, hike, cycle or swim and be physically active for at least an hour a day, or more if your health and the physical constitution allows. In case you are struggling with excess weight, you should work on removing extra kilograms as this will aid in your recovery and work benevolently on your health. If you are having problems with blood sugar levels, presuming that the sugar levels in your blood are too high, cut on white flour and sugar. Stay hydrated and drink water instead of other beverages.

What are common dietary restrictions in the renal diet?

Renal diet prescribes recommended restriction of potassium and sodium as damaged kidneys are having problems with leveling these minerals in your body. When having increased levels of potassium and sodium, even though these minerals are essential for your health and your overall well-being, more damage can be brought upon your renal system. Aside from recommending low intake of potassium and sodium, renal diet also promotes decreased consumption of phosphorus.
You may feel at the beginning of renal diet that there are too many restrictions and that these food "bans" are too difficult to follow up with, however, you can talk to your doctor about recommended dosage of sodium and potassium through your daily diet based on your health condition.

Hopefully, any doubts that you might have had about the renal diet are now all clear, while you have learned more about positive effects that this dietary regimen should have on your renal health with the ultimate goal of stopping progression of your chronic kidney's disease.
We have already placed an emphasis on how important it is for your health to cut down on potassium and sodium, however, there is another mineral that needs to be limited in your diet in order to improve your renal functions–phosphorus.

Phosphorus and How It Relates to Kidneys Disease

Renal diet prescribes careful monitoring of potassium and sodium in your body, as although essential in order for your body to be able to function properly, excess levels of these minerals can cause more health problems and bring more damage to your kidneys. The same thing goes for phosphorus levels in your body.
Phosphorus represents an essential mineral that serves the purpose of maintaining bone structure and taking care of bone cells development. Phosphorus has more roles in our organism as an essential mineral, working on connective tissue repair and enabling muscle movement. However, when concentrations of this mineral in your organism are too high as kidneys are unable to level phosphorus levels due to slow and damaged renal functions, redundant phosphorus becomes dangerous and may cause further health complications and aid in progression of your chronic kidney's disease. Once phosphorus levels in your blood have surpassed recommended concentrations, the otherwise useful

mineral becomes dangerous for your health as phosphorus then draws calcium from your bones, making the bones weak.

Common signs that appear as symptoms at kidney patients who have increased levels of phosphorus in their blood can appear in form of heart calcification, weak and easily breakable bones, muscle pain, as well as calcification of skin and joints, as well as blood vessel calcification. With high levels of phosphorus that damaged kidneys are not able to eject from your blood, calcium builds up and can affect your lungs, eyes, heart, and blood vessels, altogether bringing more damage to your renal functions that are already weakened. That is why watching out for phosphorus levels besides monitoring levels of potassium and sodium is essential for your renal health and can be easily conducted through a suitable diet such as renal diet that originally prescribes low-sodium and low-potassium intake on a daily basis.

Just as it is the case with potassium and sodium, phosphorus is a mineral found in many different food groups, which means that intake of this essential mineral can be monitored through food consumption.

Phosphorus in Food: How to Lower Phosphorus Levels Through Renal Diet

As you may monitor your intake of potassium and sodium through restricting food groups that have high concentrations of these minerals, you can likewise make sure to introduce your body to healthy levels of phosphorus with an appropriate diet. The entire philosophy of lowering phosphorus levels that should be regulated by your kidneys is to lower the intake of foods that are rich in this mineral. We don't recommend to completely let go of phosphorus-rich food groups as your body still needs phosphorus regardless of the state of your kidneys. Consult with your doctor to find out more about phosphorus levels in your blood so you would know which food you may need to give up on.

Foods that normally have high concentrations of phosphorus are meat, cheese, dairy, seeds, soda, seeds and fast foods, so you may want to watch out for these food groups and make sure that your overall consumption of protein and dairy is restricted and limited just as it is the case with foods rich in sodium and potassium.

In case phosphorus levels found in your blood are higher than recommended according to your physician you are more likely to be advised to cut on meat and dairy portions, while meat also contains high concentrations of potassium.

Best way of monitoring quantities of phosphorus, potassium and sodium you are ingesting through your everyday diet is to limit the food groups that contain high concentrations of these minerals. Beside from limiting foods that contain high levels of these minerals, you can also limit phosphorus introduced to your organism by cutting on portions that contain food that is high in phosphorus, sodium or potassium. Make sure to get familiar with which food groups contain highest concentrations of phosphorus, while eating fresh veggies and fruit may help you in case you have increased phosphorus in your blood. Food that has more than 120 mg of phosphorus per serving is considered to be high-phosphorus food, and should be introduced to your diet in limited amounts and in smaller portions, as well as it is the case with foods that are rich in potassium and sodium.

Phosphorus in Food: DO's and DON'T's

To help you follow up with food groups that are rich in phosphorus as well as foods that have low concentrations of phosphorus, we have compiled yet another grocery list that should help you with your shopping in case you need to lower quantities of phosphorus introduced to your body through food.

- **Low Phosphorus Foods (less than 120 mg per serving)**

    - Baby carrots
    - Apple
    - Figs
    - Cherries
    - Celery
    - Fruit juice - organic
    - Berry fruit such as strawberry and blueberry
    - Radishes
    - Pears
    - Cabbage
    - Cucumber
    - Snow peas
    - Cauliflower
    - Lettuce
    - Turnips
    - Most fresh veggies are low in phosphorus although you may want to watch out for veggies that are high in potassium
    - Cheese choices such as cream cheese and blue cheese—make sure that your cheese choices that are low in phosphorus are not simultaneously high in potassium and sodium
    - Pearled barley
    - Couscous

- White pasta
- White rice
- White bread and pastry

- **Food that contains high concentrations of phosphorus**

- Dark grains
- Unrefined grains
- Whole grains
- Beans of different types
- Dried vegetables
- Dried fruit
- Chocolate
- Poultry
- Beef
- Different types of fish and seafood have phosphorus concentrations above 120 mg
- Meat in general has high concentrations of phosphorus and potassium
- Most cheeses have high levels of phosphorus

Make sure to discuss a more personalized diet with your doctor, as well as take phosphate binders with every meal if prescribed. Phosphate binders are often prescribed for patients with damaged kidney function as binders are due to absorb redundant phosphate introduced to the body by ingestion. In case you are taking phosphate binders, discuss with your physician on which food groups from the provided list you should remove, increase or decrease in consumption.

Protein in Renal Diet

It may appear based on the recommendations in the book regarding protein intake that renal diet and protein don't get along that well, which is not very accurate or a fact. Renal diet promotes healthy living with low and damaged renal function, different stages of chronic kidneys disease, and has the ultimate goal to help improve renal health at patients who have been diagnosed with a kidney's disease, as well as helping prevention of chronic kidneys disease at patients with high-risk rates.

Protein is an essential nutrient that our body needs for variety of vital roles in our organism, among which is the overall ability of tissue repair and wound healing as well as "feeding" our muscle mass. Especially when some of the body functions are weak, patients may need extra protein in order to be able to recover and improve their health. However, since kidneys have the role of processing protein "leftovers", too much protein might become a problem for patients with damaged kidneys. Since kidneys are unable to remove all the waste that remains from processing protein, the body become overwhelmed with toxic waste that can't leave the body. That is actually the main reason why renal diet prescribes and recommends smaller portions of protein for renal patients and people with high risk of getting chronic kidneys disease. Of course, the relationship between renal diet and protein is complimentary, as this dietary regimen still recommends not to skip on your protein meals even in case you don't eat meat. Protein intake at renal patients is especially recommended at people who had a successful kidney transplant surgery and are in the phase of recovery where protein is of vital significance.

Based on your test results discuss with your doctor on how much protein you are allowed to have on a daily basis for more specific dietary requirements.

Renal-Friendly Protein Sources

As mentioned before, renal diet DOES prescribe lower doses of protein and smaller portions of meat for chronic kidneys disease patients, but it DOES NOT recommend complete absence of protein in your diet. Besides meat, there are plenty of protein sources that can be described as moderately friendly or completely renal diet-friendly and in compliance with the dietary requirements, while it is very important to have your daily dose of protein. As mentioned earlier in the book, recommended dose of protein for renal patients is set at 0.8 mg per one kilogram of body weight and around 1.3 mg of protein per kilogram of body weight, unless recommended otherwise by your physician.

We also mentioned protein called albumin, commonly found in our blood with the task of repairing tissue and maintaining tissue growth, which is why you shouldn't miss out on adding protein to your diet even though you need to cut down on meat portions. To keep up healthy levels of albumin and prevent further damage of your kidneys, we are recommending some top renal-friendly foods that should help you get your daily dose of protein without jeopardizing your health.

Chicken

Chicken may have extra potassium that you don't need when your renal functions are not performing well, which is why it is recommended to lower your consumption of protein. However, lean chicken meat, especially chicken breasts are especially rich in protein and has low concentration of fat, which is exactly what you want in your protein source. Avoid consuming chicken-based products in form of pre-made chicken roast found in stores, as well as processed and canned meat which is packed with potassium and sodium that you are looking to lower in your diet. One portion of chicken meat may contain up to 28 grams of protein.

Cheese

Cottage cheese might have the right amount of animal-based protein that your body needs, however, cottage cheese might have higher concentrations of sodium while it also has high levels of potassium. Try going for low-sodium cheese when looking for more protein sources other than meat. You should also note that low-sodium products such as cheese with lowered levels of this mineral, may offer increased potassium concentrations which you want to avoid unless specifically recommended by your doctor.

Eggs

You can have egg substitute with low sodium and low potassium concentrations, but you can also eat eggs as long as you don't exaggerate in quantity. The best source of clean protein for you is found in egg whites, providing you with around 7 grams of protein.

Yogurt

When substituting meat, try having Greek yogurt instead, as this dairy product is less harmful for your renal system when compared to the effects milk can leave on your health when having problems with renal functions. One serving of Greek yogurt will provide you with approximately 20 grams of animal-based protein.

- Tofu burgers

Tofu burgers and other tofu products may be a good alternative for protein sources where eating meat is not an option out of a specific reason, while a serving of tofu will provide you the same amount of protein as egg whites from one egg.

- Protein shake

Protein supplements that are compliant with renal diet and approved by your physician may represent. Protein supplements can be mixed with fruit and drinks, as well as be added to your food, which can be a great way of adding protein where there are no options for eating meat or finding protein in other food sources.

Fish

You can get up to 20 grams of protein in one serving of fish such as salmon, which actually has lower concentrations of potassium when compared to other fish.

Controlling Protein in Renal Diet

We have already made an emphasis on how important is to cut your protein portions when on renal diet while also managing to ingest enough protein so you wouldn't have further health complications.

Since you should be monitoring your protein intake carefully so you would be able to improve your overall health, we have compiled a quick checklist of things you need to look out for in order to keep your protein intake under control and at normal levels that won't put additional pressure on your vital organs.

- Protein Control Check List

- ✓ Avoid processed meat such as sausage, salami, canned meat and other meat products that may contain higher concentrations of sodium and potassium.
- ✓ Try having protein in form of meat and fish only once a day. You may choose lunch or dinner as your meat/fish meal.
- ✓ Avoid adding salt to your meat—instead use garlic powder, herbs and different safe seasonings that we have listed in our Ultimate Renal Grocery List.
- ✓ Try baking, broiling, grilling or steam cooking your meat instead of eating fried meat.
- ✓ Choose lean and fresh meat for improved health.
- ✓ Cut your protein portions.

Top Renal Food Choices

Just as there are some food groups that you should avoid consuming in order to preserve your renal health, there are certain foods that actually represent "superfoods" when following up with renal diet recommendations. We encourage you to increase your intake of these groceries as we picked top renal food choices for low and damaged kidney functions, also explaining why these foods are great for you and your renal health.

Blueberry

Blueberry is known to have amazing antioxidant properties, which means that a combination of nutrients found in this berry fruit should help you deal with toxic waste, especially in cases where your renal functions are weakened. At the same time, blueberry has low concentrations of potassium, sodium, as well as phosphorus. Antioxidant bodies contained in blueberry may help you prevent all types of cancer, as well as prevent cardiovascular disease thanks to the combination of vitamins this power fruit has.

- Red Grapes

Red grapes represent another power fruit that has low concentrations of potassium, phosphorus and sodium. Besides representing a safe source of nutrients when on renal diet, red grapes are rich in vitamin C. Red grapes also contain a certain type of antioxidants that are proven to be effective in reducing inflammation, which is another reason why red grapes should be encouraged into your diet. This fruit may also help with prevention of diabetes and heart disease.

Garlic

As advised earlier in the book, garlic makes a great substitution to salt when in need of lowering sodium levels in your body just as it is the case with renal diet. You can use garlic as a delicious substitute for salt, while also taking advantage of some amazing properties that garlic has. Garlic is a great source of vitamin B6 as well as vitamin C, while it is proven to have inflammatory properties, also working on improving your immune system. Garlic as well has low levels of sodium, phosphorus and potassium, which makes it renal-friendly.

Cabbage

Cabbage is one of the most powerful veggies that you can introduce to your everyday diet if the power of a vegetable is measured in vitamins, minerals and other essential nutrients. Besides from having low levels of potassium and other minerals that may harm your damaged renal system, cabbage is a rich source of vitamins C, K, and vitamin B. Cabbage is thus a renal-friendly food, but it also works great on your digestive health, offering fiber that good bacteria is using for food, keeping your gut health in check and clean.

- Bell Peppers

Bell peppers are another rich source of vitamin C with only half a bell pepper representing concentrations of this vitamin that are enough for your daily needs. Bell peppers also contain high concentrations of vitamin A, thus having amazing effects on your immune system, additionally packed with strong doses of antioxidants. Bell peppers are extremely welcome into renal diet, having low concentrations of potassium and sodium.

- Egg Whites

Egg whites are packed with protein that your body needs for muscle mass. Since your kidneys are having a hard time processing protein leftover that quickly turns into toxic waste, you are advised not to exaggerate with animal-based protein, however, we encourage consumption of egg whites as a clean source of pure protein. Eggs are especially recommended for dialysis patients and patients who have already had a successful kidney transplant and are in need of good protein sources. Yolks are also very nutritious and packed with protein, however, egg yolks have high doses of phosphorus as should be avoided in large quantities. Egg whites, on the other hand, have low concentrations of potassium, sodium, and phosphorus, representing one of the top renal-friendly choices.

Cauliflower

Cauliflower will probably be one of your favorite substitutes for veggies that are high in potassium, such as potatoes, while you can also use cauliflower as a substitute for rice that has lower levels of carbohydrates in case you are trying to cut on carbs. Cauliflower is low in potassium and sodium, also making a poor source of phosphorus, which makes this veggie a great source of nutrients for you. Cauliflower is also rich in vitamin K, A, and vitamin C, and represents a rich source of fiber, having anti-inflammatory properties which is great for people that need to follow the renal diet.

Cranberries

Cranberry is indeed a super fruit for people who are suffering from health conditions related to renal system and kidneys, as well as for people who have issues with urinary tract. Cranberry contains special nutrient flora that prevents different types of bacteria from remaining in the urinary tract, that way removing risk factor for urinary tract health conditions. Cranberry is also renal-friendly as it has very low concentrations of potassium, phosphorus and sodium, thus making a safe source of nutrients when on renal diet. While following the renal diet you can consume cranberry fresh, cooked, as cranberry sauce, or juiced, however, it is advised to avoid eating dried fruit—even dried cranberries.

Onion

Onion is rich in fiber which represents great food for your gastrointestinal bacteria, keeping your gut healthy and protected by the good bacteria. Besides from helping your gut work properly and keeping up the numbers of good bacteria, onions are low in potassium and sodium concentrations, as well as phosphorus levels. You can use this nutrient-rich veggie as a base for numerous different meals, while we recommend using sautéed onion with garlic and some olive oil for seasoning your meat and cooking your meals. This combination will make a tasty substitute for salt, coming with far less sodium and making a healthier option for you. Onion also has high concentrations of vitamin C and several types of vitamin B, which makes it a great source of nutrients for you and your renal health.

Pineapple

Pineapple might become your sweet escape in case you are a fan of sweets and candies, while pineapple makes a far healthier options than sugary treats. This sweet and savory fruit has low concentrations of phosphorus, potassium and sodium, and it represents a rich source of fibers and enzymes that have anti-inflammatory properties. Pineapple is also rich in different types of vitamins B, which is another reason to add this wonderous tropical fruit to your grocery list.

- Chicken Breasts

Chicken breasts represent lean meat packed with protein and is probably the best choice for your animal-based protein as long as you have chicken with no skin and as far as you manage to keep your meat portions small and moderately added to your everyday diet. Chicken breasts as almost any other type of meat contains higher doses of potassium, sodium and phosphorus, however, skinless chicken breasts prepared slow-cooked or baked with some veggies can make a great source of protein on renal diet. Make sure to skin the chicken before eating, while adding garlic and other low-sodium alternatives other than salt.

- Shiitake Mushrooms

Renal diet encourages mushrooms as an alternative protein source in case you are skipping on meat or avoid consuming meat. Shiitake mushrooms are especially welcome into your diet as this type of mushrooms has lower levels of potassium when compared to other species of mushrooms. Besides from offering useful doses of protein and less potassium, shiitake are also rich in selenium, copper and B vitamins, also having low levels of sodium.

- Arugula

Arugula is another low-potassium veggie that can come as a great substitute for greens such as kale and spinach that have higher doses of potassium, while arugula also represents a great source of vitamin K. Arugula also has important nitrates that work on lowering blood pressure, which is extremely important for renal health as high blood pressure may bring more damage to your kidneys while it also makes one of the main indicators that something is wrong with the kidneys due to increased sodium levels and other risk factors. We encourage you to use arugula as a side dish and in your salads, as well as additional source of calcium.

Some Strategies/Tips on How to Behave During a Renal Diet

If you have kidney failure, damaged kidney or symptoms of kidney problems then you must follow a renal diet. The renal diet focuses more on the foods you should avoid because they are directly detrimental to your kidney health.

The Renal diet controls your consumption of sodium, protein, potassium and phosphorous. A renal diet contributes to preventing renal failure. Below are a list of food/nutrients you should avoid preventing kidney related problems:

Phosphate: Consumption of phosphate becomes dangerous when kidney failure reaches 80% and goes to the 4th/5th stage of kidney failure. So, it is better to lower your phosphate intake by counting the calories and minerals.

Protein: Being on a renal diet, you should intake 0.75 kg protein per day. Good source of protein are eggs, milk, cheese, meat, nuts, and fish.

Potassium: After getting diagnosed, if your results show your potassium level is high in the blood, then you should restrict your potassium intake. Baked and fried potatoes are very high in potassium. Leafy greens, fruit juices are high in potassium. You can still enjoy vegetables that are low in potassium.

Sodium: Adding salt is very important in our food, but when you are suffering from kidney problems, you have to omit or minimize your salt intake. Too much sodium intake can trigger high blood pressure and fluid retention in the body. You need to find substitutes that help season your food. Herbs and spices that are extracted from plants are a good option. Using garlic, pepper, mustard can increase the taste of your food without adding any salt. Avoid artificial "salts" that are low in sodium because they are high in potassium, which is also dangerous for kidney health.

What to Eat & Avoid on a Renal Diet

The renal diet focuses on more on what not to eat to improve your kidney health. But it is also essential to know what would actually benefit a kidney patient or someone who has renal dysfunction. There should be clarity regarding how much minerals, nutrients, and fluids one can eat during a renal diet. We know renal diet endorses to limit your protein intake, but does this mean it is not essential to eat protein on a renal diet? No, you should definitely eat about 7-8 ounces of protein every single day. You should have one meal dedicated to protein which would contain 7-8 ounce.

It is essential to combat infections. It also balances muscle mass. This is a healthy way to limit your protein intake on a renal diet. The sources of protein are many, milk, egg, meat, fish, pulses, etc. There are other plant-based proteins too like soy, mushroom, etc.

You should eat fresh vegetables and fruits which would be low in sodium and fat. They should not be frozen, because in most cases, frozen ingredients have preservatives in them. Some of the frozen foods also contain seasonings too. When you are picking your vegetables, make sure to stay far away from the ones that have a large quantity of potassium. When you sit and list your ingredients, you would find more things are on the positive list than the omitted ingredients list. So, enjoy the food, enjoy the process of this diet to live a better life.

Dishes a Dialysis Patient Can Order at Restaurants

A renal patient while going through dialysis has to be very careful about what they eat or drink. But does it mean you cannot enjoy dining out? Certainly not, you can enjoy eating at restaurants, but you need to be careful about what you are ordering. There are many people who take the menu of their favorite restaurants and show it to their dietitian and the dietitian mark which dishes are safe for a dialysis patient to eat.

Usually, the dishes in any restaurants are quite high in sodium and potassium, sometime in phosphate too, while ordering you need to ask them if they can cater to your condition and make you a unique dish that is low on protein, potassium, sodium, and phosphate. Ask them to give you a dish made from fresh ingredients rather than canned ones.

Italian and Asian food are safer options than others as they have a little seasoning and there are no greasy sauces. Even if they come with sauces, ask them not to pour the sauce on your food, instead pour it on the side or in a separate bowl.

If you go to a Chinese restaurant, you can order steamed rice, egg rolls, stir fry vegetables, dim sum, etc. In Thai restaurant, chicken skewers, spring roll, pad thai noodles, grilled chicken/fish, etc. In Japanese restaurants, you can order sashimi, tempura, etc. In Italian restaurants, you can order pasta without the sauce or sauce on the side. Try to skip soups because they have a lot of flavorings.

Smart Snacking Options for Renal Patients

It is absolutely human to crave for snacks no matter what situation you are in. Even when someone is sick, they still crave for snacks. Renal patients have to stay under a renal diet 24/7 to prevent unwanted renal failure. So, how to give in to your cravings whilst being on a renal diet? This solution is simple, you need to choose a snack that is in sync with your renal diet, and that does not make your situation worse.

There are many healthy snacking options for renal patients. Your snacks have to be adequately counted where they would not cross the limit of sodium, potassium, phosphate and protein intake per day. A good renal snack should be less than 80mg phosphorous, less than 130 mg potassium.

Some patients can enjoy more than other patients, to find out how much nutrients you can consume daily, you need to check with your doctor or dietitian.

Here are a few tasty snacking options:
- One cup of Popcorn rice cereal
- Pretzels Blueberries (fresh)
- 2 Breadsticks
- ½ of a muffin
- ½ of bagel
- ½ cup sorbet
- Fruit cocktail
- 2 Fig cookies 1 apple
- Few grapes (10-15)
- Vanilla wafers
- To name a few

You should not go for snacks 5-6 times a day. Instead build a healthy snacking cycle where you only crave for it when you are actually hungry. Do not give into your snacking craving every single time you have an urge for it.

Top 10 Foods to Eat for Kidney Health

Everyone's body is different as such it would be impossible to craft an eating plan that is the best fit for everyone that has kidney disease. The list of items that you can enjoy will as a result change over time, as your kidney health progresses. There are also a few other factors that will over time affect your diet, including any chronic diseases that you may also be struggling with. By working closely with your health care providers and continuing to educate yourself, you can master the art of making healthy food choices to fit your needs and will be able to personally manage your disease with tremendous success.

The following Top 10 list is geared towards general Kidney health and not necessarily strict for patients with CKD. Here are my top 10 foods for General Kidney Health:

- Cauliflower
- Blueberries
- Buckwheat Egg
- White Sea Bass
- Olive Oil Cabbage
- Skinless Chicken
- Onion
- Red Grapes

Different stages of kidney disease. A little explanation

During this hectic time of diagnosis and management of your new lifestyle, it is helpful to explore CKD and outline a few common symptoms. CKD can be defined simply as the gradual loss of kidney function. Since the body is constantly producing waste, the kidneys play a key role in removing these toxins and keeping your system functioning properly. Tests can be done to measure the specific level of wastes in your blood and determine the level of function of your kidneys. Your doctor can figure out your kidney's filtration rate and identify your CKD stage based on this measurement.

There are five stages associated with CKD that correspond to how well your kidneys are functioning. During the early stages, people often do not experience any symptoms, and the disease can be very manageable. Kidney disease can even go undetected until it is quite advanced. Many symptoms do not begin to appear until the later stages, when toxins begin to build up in the body from damage to the kidneys. For example, itching, swelling, nausea, vomiting, or changes in urine patterns may be the result of the decreased filtration ability of these organs. That's why early diagnosis is so crucial and can result in very positive outcomes later on with regard to the disease's progression.

Although there is no cure for CKD, this disease is completely manageable. Making changes to your diet and lifestyle can help slow the progression of the disease and avoid symptoms that typically begin to emerge later on. These diet and lifestyle changes can even improve your overall health and help you manage associated conditions. As we will explore in the next few sections, there are associated diseases that may have led to CKD or perhaps were a contributing factor. When you begin making changes to your food and daily habits, you will also begin to notice improvement in these associated conditions, including hypertension and diabetes.
It is very possible to live a long, healthy, and happy life while managing this disease, and making the proper changes early on can slow the progression of any adverse symptoms for several years. I hope this book will shed this important light on you and your loved ones, so together we can make positive changes that delay the progression of CKD for a long time to come.

The "CKD 1–4 diet" can be overwhelming at first, but like anything new, once you begin to put it into practice, it will become a natural part of your lifestyle that requires little thought. The basic guidelines of the CKD 1–4 diet are restriction of protein, sodium, potassium, phosphorus, and in some cases, fluids. Based on your blood-work results and other factors, your dietitian and/or health care provider can create an individualized diet prescription for you. The rest is up to you. In fact, how well you comply with these dietary restrictions has enormous influence over the rate of disease progression.

This book focuses on a wide variety of foods that can be included in the CKD 1–4 diet. It provides examples of daily meal plans that are easy and quick to prepare, corresponding shopping lists, and 151 practical recipes to suit everyone's tastes. We all have good and bad days, and diet slipups may happen. Remember, it's not about perfection but what you do most of the time that matters!

STAGES OF CKD

Stage 1: Slight kidney damage, and usually no symptoms. (eGFR > 90 mL)
Stage 2: Mild damage in kidneys (eGFR = 60–89 mL)
Stage 3: Moderate damage in kidneys (eGFR = 30–59 mL)
Stage 4: Severe damage in kidneys (eGFR = 15–29 mL)
Stage 5: Kidney failure/End-stage CKD (GFR < 15 mL)

The Role of Phosphorous in Our Body

Phosphorous contribute to keep our bone strong and develop it. Phosphorous helps in muscle movement, develops the connective tissue and organs. While we eat food that contains phosphorous, the small intestines store it to develop our bones. A well-functioning kidney can get rid of the extra phosphorous in the body, but a damaged one cannot do so. So renal patients have to watch how much phosphorous they are consuming.

As phosphorous helps to develop bones, it can also weaken the bones by extracting calcium from it if too much phosphorous is consumed. The calcium removed from the bones gets deposited to blood vessels, heart, eyes, and lungs which can cause severe health problems.

To keep the balance of phosphorous for a renal patient, the proper knowledge of high phosphorous food is required. Red meat is very high in phosphorous. Milk is very high in phosphorous. Fast food like burgers, pizzas, fries is high in phosphorous. Fizzy drinks that are colored are high in phosphorous. Canned fish and seeds are quite high in phosphorous.

Packaged food or canned food is often high in phosphorous. Read the labels before you purchase any canned goods from the supermarket. Phosphorous binders are excellent way to keep your phosphorous intake to a minimum. If you ask you your dietitian, they will give you an excellent phosphorous binder, which you can follow to keep track of how much you can and should consume.

The Role of Potassium in Our Body

Potassium maintains the balance of electrolyte and fluid in our bloodstream. It also regulates our heartbeat and contributes to our muscle function. Potassium can be found in many fruits, vegetables, and meat it also exists in our own body. A healthy kidney keeps the required potassium in our body and removes the excess through urine.

A damaged kidney is not capable of removing potassium anymore. Therefore, is it essential for a renal patient to watch how much potassium they are consuming. Hyperkalemia is a condition when you have too much potassium in the blood. Hyperkalemia can cause slow pulse, weak muscles, irregular heart rate, heart attack, and even death.

To control your potassium intake on a daily basis, count every ingredient's potassium level. A renal expert dietitian would be helpful to consult as they know which ingredient would work best for your condition. There are seasonings available in the super-shops which are high in potassium, avoid these items. Food like avocado, beans, spinach, fish, bananas, and potatoes are very high in potassium. Even if you are eating these ingredients, try to divide the serving in half and eat a small serving.

Do not eat these high potassium ingredients every single day. There are much low potassium foods available, pick them when you are making your meal plan. Fresh ingredients are always better than the frozen kind. To keep track of your potassium intake throughout the day, keep a personal food journal where you can input everything and reflect when you need to.

The Role of Sodium in our Body

A renal patient has to cut down on sodium and potassium on a daily basis in order to keep their kidney at rest. Before you limit your sodium and potassium intake, you should know what role they play in our body. Sodium and salt are not interchangeable. People have the misconception that the only salt contains sodium, but there are natural foods that are high on sodium too. Salt is a mixture of chloride and sodium. Canned food and processed food have a large amount of sodium in them. A renal patient has to consider that fact that natural food can contain sodium too.

Our body has three significant electrolytes, sodium, potassium and chloride. Sodium regulates blood vessels and blood pressure, regulates muscle contraction, nerve function, regulates the acid balance in the blood, and keep the balance of fluid in the body! The kidney usually excretes the toxin in our body, but a damaged kidney cannot get rid of the extra sodium in our body.

So, when a renal patient consumes too much sodium, it gets stored in the blood vessels and bloodstream. This storage of sodium can lead to feeling thirsty all the time. This is a bit problematic as a kidney patient has to limit their fluid intake. It can cause edema, high blood pressure, breathless, and even heart failure. So, a renal patient must always limit their sodium intake. The average limit is 150 mg per snacks and 400 mg per meal.

How to Manage and Improve Kidney Health

Patients who struggle from kidney health issues, going through kidney dialysis and have renal impairments need to not only go through medical treatment but also change their eating habit, lifestyle to make the situation better. Many researches have been done on this, and the conclusion is food has a lot to do with how your kidney functions and its overall health.

The first thing to changing your lifestyle is knowing about how your kidney functions and how different food can trigger different reactions in the kidney function. There are certain nutrients that affect your kidney directly. Nutrients like sodium, protein, phosphate, and potassium are the risky ones. You do not have to omit them altogether from your diet, but you need to limit or minimize their intake as much as possible. You cannot leave out essential nutrient like protein from your diet, but you need to count how much protein you are having per day. This is essential in order to keep balance in your muscles and maintaining a good functioning kidney.

A vast change in kidney patients is measuring how much fluid they are drinking. This is a crucial change in every kidney patient, and you must adapt to this new eating habit. Too much water or any other form of liquid can disrupt your kidney function. How much fluid you can consume depends on the condition of your kidney. Most people assign separate bottles for them so that they can measure how much they have drunk and how much more they can drink throughout the day.

Chapter 2: THE RECIPES

Breakfast Recipes

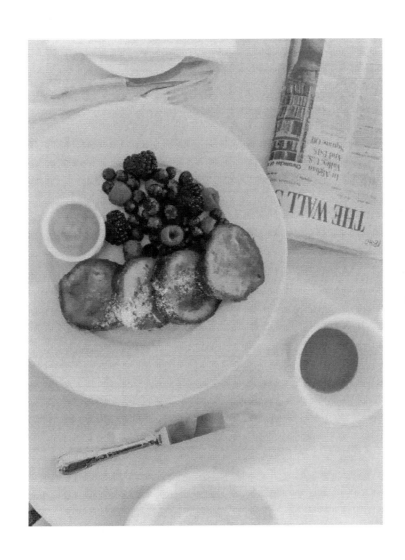

1. Egg White and Pepper Omelet

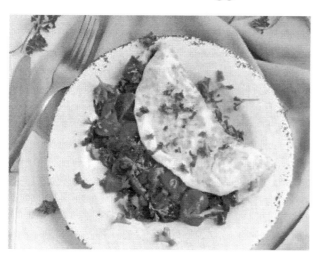

COOKING TIME: 5 MIN
DESCRIPTION

A low-calorie omelet recipe with red bell peppers that you can make in under 5 minutes with just 5 ingredients. Feel free to enhance its taste with paprika or Mexican spices.

INGREDIENTS FOR 1-2 SERVINGS
- 4 egg whites, lightly beaten
- 1 red bell pepper, diced
- 1 tsp. of paprika
- 2 tbsp. of olive oil
- ½ tsp of salt
- Pepper

METHOD
1. In a shallow pan (around 8 inches), heat the olive oil and sauté the bell peppers until softened.
2. Add the egg whites and the paprika and fold the edges into the fluid center with a spatula and let omelet cook until eggs are fully opaque and solid.
3. Season with salt and pepper.

Serve: 3

NUTRITIONAL INFORMATION (Per Serving)
- Calories: 165 kcal
- Carbohydrate: 3.8g
- Protein: 9.2g
- Sodium: 797mg
- Potassium: 193mg
- Phosphorus: 202.5mg
- Dietary Fiber: 0.7g
- Fat: 15.22g

Kidney Disease Stage: 2

2. Blueberry Smoothie Bowl

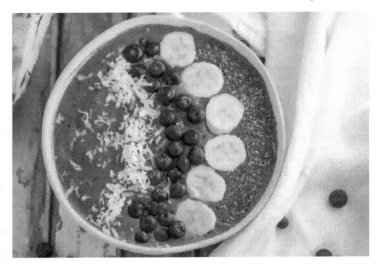

COOKING TIME: 1 MIN
DESCRIPTION
An Instagram worthy purple smoothie bowl made with frozen blueberries that are fortified with antioxidants. Plus, it counts less than 150mg of potassium and phosphorus per serving.

INGREDIENTS FOR 1 SERVING
- ½ cup of frozen blueberries
- ½ cup of vanilla flavored almond milk
- 1 tbsp. of agave syrup
- 1 tsp. of chia seeds

METHOD
1. Combine everything except for the chia seeds in the blender until smooth. You should end up with a thick smoothie paste.
2. Transfer into a cereal bowl and top with chia seeds on top.

NUTRITIONAL INFORMATION (Per Serving)
- Calories: 278.5 kcal
- Carbohydrate: 38.72g
- Protein: 1.3g
- Sodium: 76.33mg
- Potassium: 229.1mg
- Phosphorus: 59.2mg
- Dietary Fiber: 7.4g
- Fat: 6g

Kidney Disease Stage 1

3. Turkey Breakfast Sausage

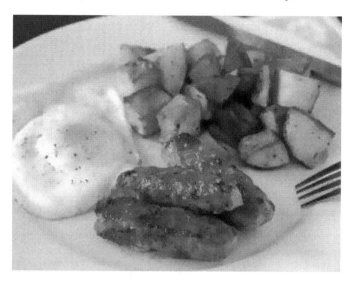

COOKING TIME: 6 MIN
DESCRIPTION

Fancy a quick sausage for breakfast or brunch? Try this low potassium breakfast sausage with turkey and spices-feel free to serve this with cornbread and apple sauce.

INGREDIENTS FOR 12 SERVINGS

(12 patties per recipe)
- 1 pound of lean ground turkey
- 1 tsp. of fennel seed
- ¼ tsp. garlic powder
- ¼ tsp. onion powder
- ¼ tsp. salt
- 2 tbsp. of vegetable oil
- Pepper

METHOD
1. Combine all the ingredients apart from the vegetable oil in a mixing bowl.
2. Form into long and flat (around 4 inch-long) patties.
3. Heat the vegetable oil in a medium frying pan.
4. Add 3-4 patties at a time and cook for approx. 3 minutes on each side. Repeat until you cook all patties.
5. Serve warm.

NUTRITIONAL INFORMATION (Per Serving)
- Calories: 74kcal
- Carbohydrate: 0.1g
- Protein: 7g
- Sodium: 121.9mg
- Potassium: 89.5mg
- Phosphorus: 75mg
- Dietary Fiber: 0g
- Fat: 5.16g

Kidney Disease Stage 2

4. Italian Apple Fritters

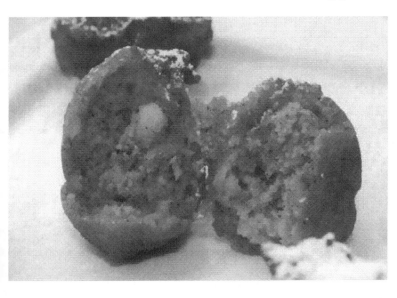

COOKING TIME: 8 MIN

DESCRIPTION

A quick apple fritter recipe with corn flour batter that is great for breakfast and dessert too. Make this preferably in a deep fryer and enjoy hot as it will lose its crisp after a few minutes.

INGREDIENTS FOR 4 SERVINGS

- 2 large apples, seeded, peeled and thickly sliced in round circles
- 3 tbsp. of corn flour
- ½ tsp. of water
- 1 tsp. of sugar
- 1 tsp. of cinnamon
- Vegetable oil (for frying)
- Sprinkle of icing sugar or honey

METHOD

1. In a small bowl, combine the corn flour, water and sugar to make your batter
2. Deep the apple rounds into the cornflour mix.
3. Heat enough vegetable oil to cover half of the pan's surface over medium to high heat.
4. Add the apple rounds into the pan and cook until golden brown.
5. Transfer into a shallow dish with absorbing paper on top and sprinkle with a bit of cinnamon and icing sugar.

NUTRITIONAL INFORMATION (Per Serving)

- Calories: 183 kcal
- Carbohydrate: 17.9g
- Protein: 0.3g
- Sodium: 2g
- Potassium: 100mg
- Phosphorus: 12.5mg
- Dietary Fiber: 1.4g
- Fat: 14.17g

Kidney Disease Stage 3

5. Tofu and Mushroom Scramble

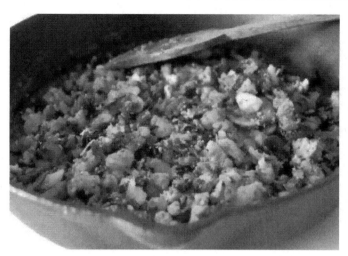

COOKING TIME: 8 MIN
DESCRIPTION

A hearty mushroom scramble recipe for vegans or fans of earthy mushroom flavors enhanced by a fine blend of exotic spices. Great for breakfast or a delicious savory brunch.

INGREDIENTS FOR 2 SERVINGS

- ½ cup of sliced white mushrooms
- ⅓ cup of medium-firm tofu, crumbled
- 1 tbsp. of chopped shallots
- ⅓ tsp. turmeric
- 1 tsp. of cumin
- ⅓ tsp. of smoked paprika
- ½ tsp. of garlic salt
- Pepper
- 3 tbsp. of vegetable oil

METHOD

1. Heat the oil in a medium frying pan and saute the sliced mushrooms with the shallots until softened (around 3-4 minutes) over medium to high heat.
2. Add the tofu pieces and toss in the spices and the garlic salt. Toss lightly until tofu and mushrooms are nicely combined together.
3. Serve warm.

NUTRITIONAL INFORMATION (Per Serving)

- Calories: 220 kcal
- Carbohydrate: 2.59g
- Protein: 3.2g
- Sodium: 288 mg
- Potassium: 133.5mg
- Phosphorus: 68.5mg
- Dietary Fiber: 1.7g
- Fat: 23.7g

Kidney Disease Stage 3

6. Sunny Pineapple Breakfast Smoothie

COOKING TIME: 1 MIN
DESCRIPTION

A sunny and bright breakfast smoothie with the sweet and sour goodness of pineapple blended with a hint of ginger for that zingy fresh taste.

INGREDIENTS FOR 1 SERVING.
- ½ cup of frozen pineapple chunks
- ⅔ cup almond milk
- ½ tsp. of ginger powder
- 1 tbsp. of agave syrup

METHOD
1. Blend everything together in a blender until nice and smooth (around 30 seconds).
2. Transfer into a tall glass or mason jar.
3. Serve and enjoy.

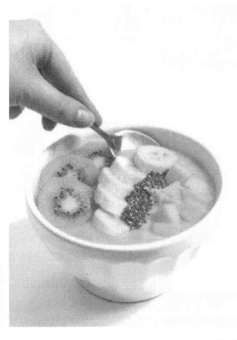

NUTRITIONAL INFORMATION (Per Serving)
- Calories: 186kcal
- Carbohydrate: 43.7g
- Protein: 2.28g
- Sodium: 130mg
- Potassium: 135mg
- Phosphorus: 18mg
- Dietary Fiber: 2.4g
- Fat: 2.3g

Kidney Disease Stage 2

7. Puff Oven Pancakes

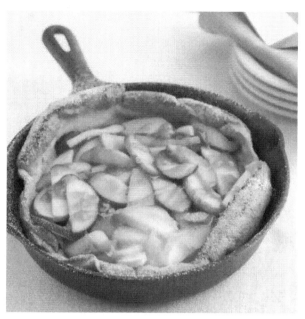

COOKING TIME: 30 MIN

DESCRIPTION

A crunchy oven pancake recipe with rice flour that is very low in potassium and phosphorus. Try this if you want something crunchy and interesting compared to ordinary pancakes.

INGREDIENTS FOR 4 SERVINGS
- 2 large eggs.
- ½ cup of rice flour
- ½ cup of rice milk
- 2 tbsp. of unsalted butter
- ⅛ tsp. of salt

METHOD
1. Preheat the oven at 400F/190C.
2. Grease a 10-inch skillet or Pyrex with the butter and heat in the oven until it melts.
3. In a mixing bowl, beat the eggs and whisk in the rice milk, flour and salt until smooth.
4. Take off the skillet or pie dish from the oven.
5. Transfer directly the batter into the skillet and put back in the oven for 25-30 minutes.
6. Place in a serving dish and cut into 4 portions.
7. Serve hot with honey or icing sugar on top.

NUTRITIONAL INFORMATION (Per Serving)
- Calories: 159.75kcal
- Carbohydrate: 17g
- Protein: 5g
- Sodium: 120g
- Potassium: 52mg
- Phosphorus: 66.25mg
- Dietary Fiber: 0.5g
- Fat: 9g

8. Savory Muffins with Protein

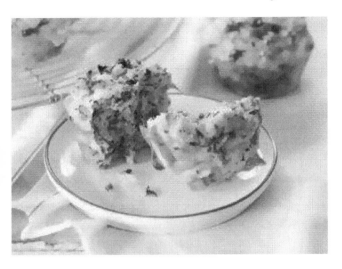

COOKING TIME 35 MIN
DESCRIPTION

A great alternative to sweet and tangy blueberry muffins. This savory muffin recipe is great alone or as a part of your breakfast. You can take it with some bacon or homemade sausage on the side and it will be delicious.

INGREDIENTS FOR 12 SERVINGS
- 2 cups of corn flakes
- ½ cup of unfortified almond milk
- 4 large eggs
- 2 tbsp. of olive oil
- 1/2 cup of almond milk
- 1 medium white onion, sliced
- 1 cup of plain Greek yogurt
- ¼ cup pecans, chopped
- 1 tbsp. of mixed seasoning blend e.g. Mrs. dash

METHOD
1. Preheat the oven at 350F/180C.
2. Heat the olive oil in the pan. Saute the onions with the pecans and seasoning blend for a couple of minutes.
3. Add the rest of ingredients and toss well.
4. Split the mixture into 12 small muffin cups (lightly greased) and bake for 30-35 minutes or until an inserted knife or toothpick is coming out clean.
5. Serve warm or keep at room temperature for a couple of days.

NUTRITIONAL INFORMATION (Per Serving)
- Calories: 106.58kcal
- Carbohydrate: 8.20g
- Protein: 4.77g
- Sodium: 51.91mg

- Potassium: 87.83 mg
- Phosphorus: 49.41 mg
- Dietary Fiber: 0.58 g
- Fat: 5 g

Kidney Disease Stage 2

9. European Pancakes

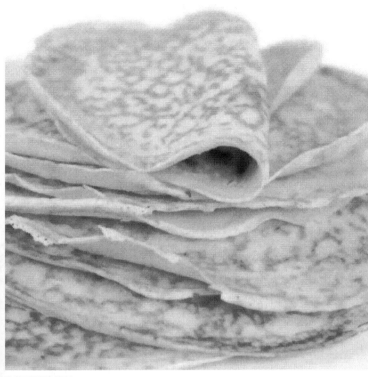

COOKING TIME: 20 MIN
DESCRIPTION
European pancakes, most favored by the French and the Germans are thin and soft and make an excellent base for other dishes-both savory and sweet. If you are making these for breakfast, top them with some fresh strawberries and honey for a low potassium sweet treat.

INGREDIENTS FOR 10 SERVINGS

(20 pancakes)

- 2/3 cups of all-purpose flour
- 4 large eggs
- 2 tbsp. of sugar
- ½ tsp. of lemon zest
- 1 cup of low-fat milk
- ¼ tsp. of vanilla extract

METHOD
1. In a medium bowl, mix the flour with the sugar. Whisk in the eggs and combine well.
2. Add the milk, vanilla, and lemon zest to the mix and whisk well.
3. Spray a small 8-10 inch pan with cooking spray and pour around 4 tbsp. of the mixture and distribute evenly by tilting the pan from one side to another.
4. Cook until the batter is solid and light golden brown (around 50 seconds on each side). Flip.
5. Repeat the above two steps until all the batter has finished.

NUTRITIONAL INFORMATION (Per Serving)
- Calories: 74kcal
- Carbohydrate: 10g
- Protein: 4g
- Sodium: 39mg
- Potassium: 73mg
- Phosphorus: 73mg
- Dietary Fiber: 0.2g
- Fat: 2g

10. Puffy French Toast

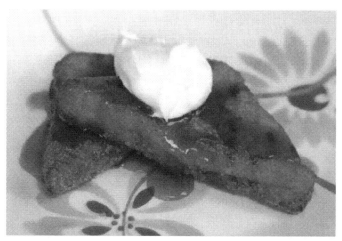

COOKING TIME: 8 MIN
DESCRIPTION

An easy French toast recipe that is dairy-free for lower amounts of phosphorus. Made in the pan and finished in the oven for an extra puffy result.

INGREDIENTS FOR 4 SERVINGS
- 4 slices of white bread, cut in half diagonally
- 3 whole eggs and 1 egg white
- 1 cup of plain almond milk
- 2 tbsp. of canola oil
- 1 tsp. of cinnamon

METHOD
1. Preheat your oven to 400F/180C
2. Beat together the eggs with the almond milk.
3. Heat the oil in a pan.
4. Dip each bread slice/triangle into the egg and almond milk mixture.
5. Fry in the pan until golden brown on each side.
6. Place the toasts in a baking dish and let cook in the oven for another 5 minutes.
7. Serve warm and drizzle with some honey, icing sugar, or cinnamon on top.

NUTRITIONAL INFORMATION (Per Serving)
- Calories: 293.75kcal
- Carbohydrate: 25.3g
- Protein: 9.27g
- Sodium: 211g
- Potassium: 97mg
- Phosphorus: 165mg
- Dietary Fiber: 12.3g
- Fat: 16.50g

Kidney Disease Stage 2

11. Vegetable Rice Casserole

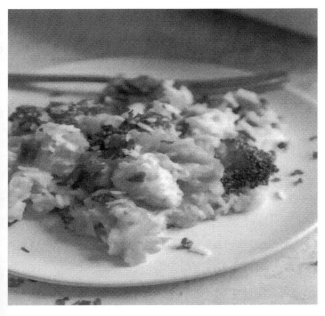

SERVES 4
PREP TIME: 10 MINUTES
COOK TIME: 50 MINUTES

LOW FAT Vegetarian dishes do not have to be complicated to be delicious. People often underestimate the unfussy recipes—there's no need to sprout your own alfalfa or press your own tofu. This recipe makes that point, with rice, vegetables, and a little sprinkle of cheese, which combine to create a perfect midweek meal or quick lunch when you need a little extra energy. Have some fun testing out all types of vegetables for different variations.

INGREDIENTS
- 1 teaspoon of olive oil
- ½ small sweet onion, chopped
- ½ teaspoon of minced garlic
- ½ cup of chopped red bell pepper
- ¼ cup of grated carrot
- 1 cup of white basmati rice
- 2 cups of water
- ¼ cup of grated Parmesan cheese
- Freshly ground black pepper

METHOD
1. Preheat the oven to 350°f.
2. In a medium skillet over medium-high heat, heat the olive oil.
3. Add the onion and garlic, and sauté until softened, about 3 minutes.
4. Transfer the vegetables to a 9-by-9-inch baking dish, and stir in the rice and water.
5. Cover the dish and bake until the liquid is absorbed 35 to 40 minutes.
6. Sprinkle the cheese on top and bake an additional 5 minutes to melt.
7. Season the casserole with pepper, and serve.

Substitution tip: Not surprisingly, the cheesy topping on this casserole elevates it to a truly sublime experience. You can also try feta, Cheddar cheese, and goat cheese for different tastes and textures.

NUTRITIONAL INFO

- PER SERVING Calories: 224 Total fat: 3g
- Saturated fat: 1g
- Cholesterol: 6mg
- Sodium: 105mg
- Carbohydrates: 41g
- Fiber: 2g
- Phosphorus: 118mg
- Potassium: 176mg
- Protein: 6g

Kidney Disease Stage 1

12. Egg Fried Rice

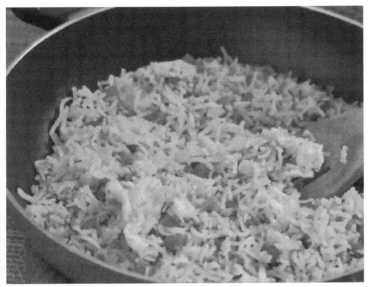

SERVES 6
PREP TIME: 10 MINUTES
COOK TIME: 20 MINUTES

This robust version of the familiar restaurant fare is more Indonesian and is close to a traditional dish called nasi goreng (fried rice), which uses limited oil and includes fresh vegetables and eggs. The egg in nasi goreng is often fried sunny-side up and placed over the finished rice, but as is directed here, scrambled works well too.

INGREDIENTS
- 1 tablespoon of olive oil
- 1 tablespoon of grated peeled fresh ginger
- 1 teaspoon of minced garlic
- 1 cup of chopped carrots
- 1 scallion, white and green parts, chopped
- 2 tablespoons of chopped fresh cilantro
- 4 cups of cooked rice
- 1 tablespoon of low-sodium soy sauce
- 4 eggs, beaten

METHOD
1. In a large skillet over medium-high heat, heat the olive oil.
2. Add the ginger and garlic, and sauté until softened, about 3 minutes.
3. Add the carrots, scallion, and cilantro, and sauté until tender, about 5 minutes.
4. Stir in the rice and soy sauce, and sauté until the rice is heated through about 5 minutes.
5. Move the rice over to one side of the skillet, and pour the eggs into the empty space.
6. Scramble the eggs, then mix them into the rice.
7. Serve hot.

Low-sodium tip: Soy sauces, even low-sodium versions, are very salty. If you have the time, making your own substitution sauce is simple and effective, even if it does not taste quite the same. There are many versions of this diet-friendly sauce online, with ingredients like vinegar, molasses, garlic, and herbs.

NUTRITIONAL INFO
- PER SERVING Calories: 204 Total fat: 6g
- Saturated fat: 1g
- Cholesterol: 141mg
- Sodium: 223mg
- Carbohydrates: 29g
- Fiber: 1g
- Phosphorus: 120mg
- Potassium: 147mg
- Protein: 8g

Kidney Disease Stage 5

13. Mushroom Rice Noodles

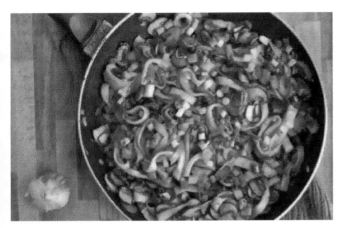

SERVES 4
PREP TIME: 15 MINUTES
COOK TIME: 15 MINUTES

LOW PROTEIN LOW FAT Rice noodles come in an assortment of types and are the foundation for many classic Asian dishes such as pad Thai and pho. You will be confronted by packages of Asian noodles when trying to pick out the ones for this recipe, with options such as udon, soba, and lo mein. Look for plain rice noodles that are transparent and about ¼ inch wide. If you get the other variations, then the nutrition data will change, because they have added ingredients like buckwheat.

INGREDIENTS
- 4 cups of rice noodles
- 2 teaspoons of toasted sesame oil
- 2 cups of sliced wild mushrooms
- 2 teaspoons of minced garlic
- 1 red bell pepper, sliced
- 1 yellow bell pepper, sliced
- 1 carrot, julienned
- 2 scallions, white and green parts, sliced
- 1 tablespoon of low-sodium soy sauce

METHOD
1. Prepare the rice noodles according to the package instructions and set them aside.
2. In a large skillet over medium-high heat, heat the sesame oil.

3. Sauté the red bell pepper, yellow bell pepper, carrot, and scallions until tender, about 5 minutes.
4. Stir in the soy sauce and rice noodles, and toss to coat.
5. Serve.

Low-sodium tip Liquid aminos or coconut aminos—a sauce usually shelved near the soy sauce in supermarkets—is a reasonable substitute for soy sauce, at about 360 mg per tablespoon. Regular soy sauce has approximately 920 mg of sodium per tablespoon and low-sodium soy sauce has approximately 575 mg per tablespoon.

NUTRITIONAL INFO
- PER SERVING Calories: 163
- Total fat: 2g
- Saturated fat: 0g
- Cholesterol: 0mg
- Sodium: 199mg
- Carbohydrates: 33g
- Fiber: 2g
- Phosphorus: 69mg
- Potassium: 200mg
- Protein: 2g

Kidney Disease Stage 4

14. Mixed Vegetable Barley

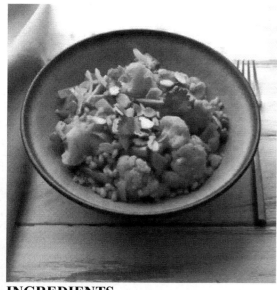

SERVES 6
PREP TIME: 15 MINUTES
COOK TIME: 35 MINUTES

LOW PROTEIN LOW FAT Barley is a cereal grain often found in soups because it adds substance, thickens the broth a little, and has a pleasing chewy texture. Very high in manganese, molybdenum, selenium, and fiber, barley is a good choice for regulating the digestive system and lowering cholesterol, as well as reducing the risk of cardiovascular disease. Either pearl barley or pot barley will yield the best results in this recipe.

INGREDIENTS

- 1 tablespoon of olive oil
- 1 medium sweet onion, chopped
- 2 teaspoons of minced garlic
- 2 cups of fresh cauliflower florets
- 1 red bell pepper, diced
- 1 carrot, sliced
- ½ cup of barley
- ½ cup of white rice
- 2 cups of water
- 1 tablespoon of minced fresh parsley

METHOD

1. In a large skillet over medium-high heat, heat the olive oil.
2. Add the onion and garlic, and sauté until softened, about 3 minutes.
3. Stir in the cauliflower, bell pepper, and carrot, and sauté for 5 minutes.
4. Stir in the barley, rice, and water and bring to a boil.
5. Reduce the heat to low, cover, and simmer until the liquid is absorbed and the barley and rice are tender about 25 minutes.

6. Serve topped with the parsley.

Cooking tip: You can bake this dish in the oven rather than cooking it on the stove and set it up completely the night before. Just transfer the sautéed vegetables to an 8-by-8-inch casserole dish and stir in the barley, rice, and water. Store in the refrigerator until ready to bake.

NUTRITIONAL INFO
- PER SERVING Calories: 156
- Total fat: 3g
- Saturated fat: 0g
- Cholesterol: 0mg
- Sodium: 16mg
- Carbohydrates: 30g
- Fiber: 4g Phosphorus: 83mg
- Potassium: 220mg Protein: 4g

Kidney Disease Stage 5

15. Spicy Sesame Tofu

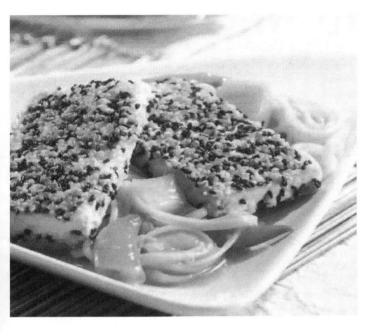

SERVES 6
PREP TIME: 15 MINUTES
COOK TIME: 10 MINUTES

LOW PROTEIN LOW FAT Dedicated vegetarians sometimes walk right past the tofu display in the supermarket because they have no idea how to prepare these blocks of pressed soy. Tofu is made in a similar technique as cheese, so you can purchase tofu from soft all the way to extra firm, depending on how much liquid has been pressed out. Tofu is an amazing ingredient because it soaks up whatever flavors you add to it, and it can cook up crispy and firm. The sesame, ginger, soy sauce, and hot red pepper flakes in this dish combine to create a truly sublime blend for infusing the tofu.

INGREDIENTS
- 1 tablespoon toasted sesame oil
- 1 tablespoon grated peeled fresh ginger
- 2 teaspoons minced garlic
- 2 red bell peppers, thinly sliced
- 1 (14-ounce) package extra-firm tofu, drained and cut into 1-inch cubes
- 2 cups quartered bok choy
- 2 scallions, white and green parts, cut thinly on a bias
- 3 tablespoons low-sodium soy sauce
- 2 tablespoons freshly squeezed lime juice
- Pinch red pepper flakes
- 2 tablespoons chopped fresh cilantro
- 2 tablespoons toasted sesame seeds

METHOD

In a large skillet over medium-high heat, heat the sesame oil.

Add the ginger and garlic, and sauté until softened, about 3 minutes.

Stir in the bell peppers and tofu, and gently sauté for about 3 minutes.

Add the bok choy and scallions, and sauté until the bok choy is wilted about 3 minutes.

Add the soy sauce, lime juice, and red pepper flakes and toss to coat.

Serve topped with the cilantro and sesame seeds.

Low-sodium tip: Almost all the sodium in this dish comes from the soy sauce, so reducing it or omitting it will significantly drop the amount of sodium per serving. The taste of the recipe will not be as strong but using just 1 tablespoon of soy sauce in this recipe will create a serving with about 160 mg sodium.

NUTRITIONAL INFO
PER SERVING Calories: 80
Total fat: 3g
Saturated fat: 0g
Cholesterol: 0mg
Sodium: 503mg
Carbohydrates: 4g
Fiber: 1g
Phosphorus: 88mg
Potassium: 165mg
Protein: 6g

Kidney Disease Stage 5

Lunch Recipes

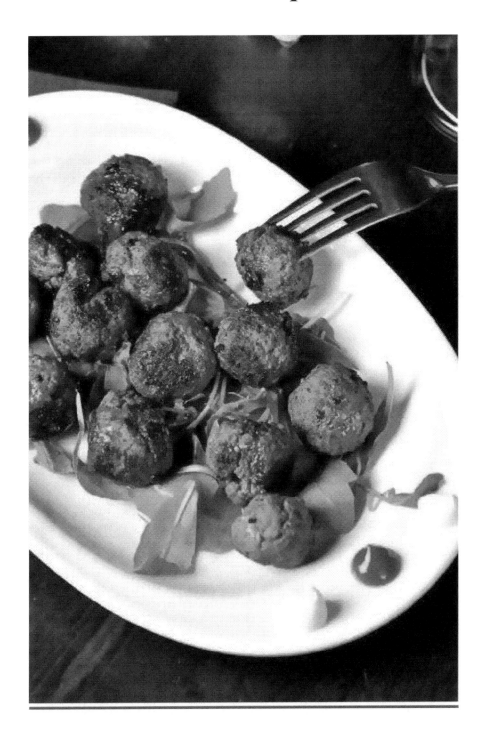

16. Creamy Chicken with Cider

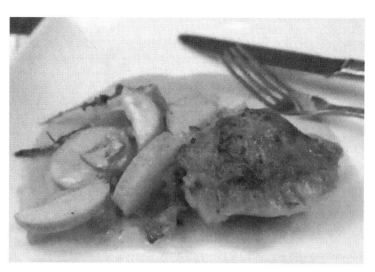

COOKING TIME: 25 MINUTES

DESCRIPTION

An easy 4-ingredient recipe that is full of flavor and is ready in under 30 minutes. Great as a family lunch on weekends or even as a hearty guest dish. It has a light gravy sauce for that extra dose of flavor.

INGREDIENTS FOR 8 SERVINGS:
- 4 bone-in chicken breasts
- 2 tbsp. of lightly salted butter
- ¾ cup of apple cider vinegar
- ⅔ cup of rich unsweetened coconut milk or cream
- Kosher pepper

METHOD
1. Melt the butter in a skillet over medium heat.
2. Season the chicken with the pepper and add to the skillet. Cook over low heat for approx. 20 minutes.
3. Remove the chicken from the heat and set aside in a dish.
4. In the same skillet, add the cider and bring to a boil until most of it has evaporated.
5. Add the coconut cream and let cook for 1 minute until slightly thickened.
6. Pour the cider cream over the cooked chicken and serve.

NUTRITIONAL INFORMATION (Per Serving)
- Calories: 86.76kcal
- Carbohydrate: 1.88g
- Protein: 1.5g
- Sodium: 93.52mg
- Potassium: 74.65mg
- Phosphorus: 36.54mg
- Dietary Fiber: 0.1g
- Fat: 8.21g

Kidney Disease Stage 3

17.   Easy and Fast Mac-n-Cheese

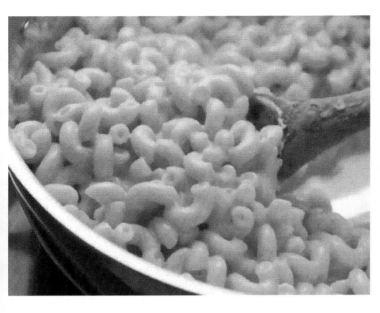

COOKING TIME: 8-10 MINUTES
DESCRIPTION

Mac-n-cheese is favorite soul food for kids and adults alike. It's not what we call "healthy" as it is loaded with a high amount of carbs but when on a renal diet, this is fine as it is very low in potassium and phosphorus.

INGREDIENTS FOR 4 SERVINGS
- 1 cup of dry elbow macaroni pasta
- ½ cup of mild cheddar cheese
- 3 cups of water
- 1 tsp. of unsalted butter
- ½ tsp. of dry mustard powder
- ½ tsp. of paprika

METHOD
1. Boil the elbow macaroni in boiling water for 7-8 minutes (or until soft).
2. Drain all the water out and transfer it in the bowl.
3. Add the butter cheese, mustard, and paprika while the pasta is still hot, toss and serve.

NUTRITIONAL INFORMATION (Per Serving)
- Calories: 231.68kcal
- Carbohydrate: 32.65g
- Protein: 9.74g
- Sodium: 107.25mg
- Potassium: 29.52mg
- Phosphorus: 159.93mg
- Dietary Fiber: 0.12g
- Fat: 7.2g

Kidney Disease Stage 2

18. Exotic Palabok

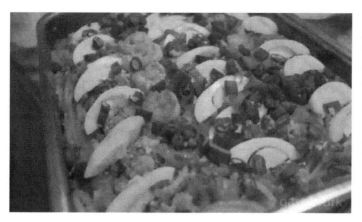

COOKING TIME: 12-15 MINUTES
DESCRIPTION

A delicious recipe from the Philippines that combines the flavors of rice noodles and shrimp.

INGREDIENTS FOR 6 SERVINGS
- 12 oz. rice noodles.
- 1 ½ cups of medium shrimp, peeled and deveined
- ⅔ cup of white onion, chopped
- 1 spring onion, sliced
- 3 tbsp. of canola oil
- 1-pound, lean ground turkey
- 2 cups of firm tofu, chopped
- 2 packs of shrimp or ordinary gravy mix
- 5 hard-boiled eggs
- 1 lemon
- ½ cup of pork rinds (optional)

METHOD
1. Boil rice noodles until nice and soft. Keep aside.
2. Boil the peeled shrimp for 2-3 minutes in a pot with plain water.
3. In a wok or shallow pan, saute the garlic and onion with the oil. Add the ground turkey, tofu, and shrimps.
4. Dissolve the gravy mix in water or as per package instructions.
5. Combine the rice noodles, tofu, onions, and the gravy mix with ½ cup of pork rind (optional).
6. Slice the egg and lemons.
7. Serve with egg and lemons on top.

NUTRITIONAL INFORMATION (Per Serving)
- Calories: 305 kcal
- Carbohydrate: 39.14g
- Protein: 17.6g
- Sodium: 536mg

- Potassium: 243.52 mg
- Phosphorus: 180.41mg
- Dietary Fiber: 0.9g

Kidney Disease Stage 4

19. Vegetarian Gobi Curry

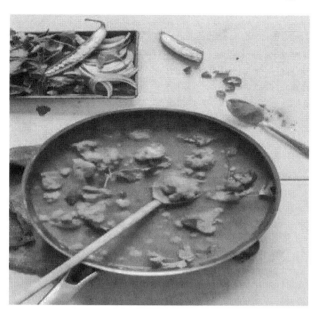

COOKING TIME: 15 MINUTES

DESCRIPTION

An ethnic Indian recipe that comes from the Gobi Desert area with a creamy and spicy flavor and texture that is a comfort for everyone. Vegetarians will love this recipe, as it's quite delicious and filling.

INGREDIENTS

- 2 cups of cauliflower florets
- 2 tbsp. of unsalted butter
- 1 medium dry white onion, thinly chopped
- ½ cup of green peas (frozen if wish)
- 1 tsp. of fresh ginger, chopped
- 1/2 tsp. of turmeric
- 1 tsp of garam masala
- ¼ tsp. cayenne pepper
- 1 tbsp. of water

METHOD

1. Heat a skillet over medium heat with the butter and sauté the onions until caramelized (golden brown).
2. Add the spices e.g. ginger, garam masala turmeric, and cayenne.
3. Add the cauliflower and the (frozen) peas and stir.
4. Add the water and cover with a lid. Reduce the heat to a low temperature and let cook covered for 10 minutes.
5. Serve with white rice.

NUTRITIONAL INFORMATION (Per Serving)

- Calories: 91.04kcal
- Carbohydrate: 7.3g
- Protein: 2.19g
- Sodium: 39.38mg
- Potassium: 209.58mg
- Phosphorus: 42mg
- Dietary Fiber: 3g
- Fat: 6.4g

Kidney Disease Stage 2

20. Marinated Shrimp and Pasta

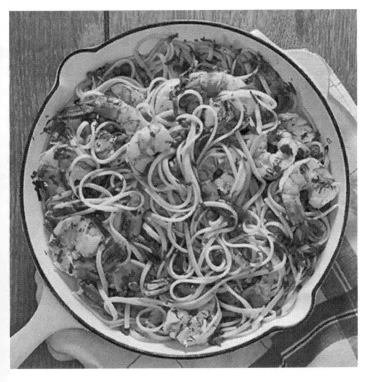

COOKING TIME: 10 MINUTES
DESCRIPTION

A hearty recipe that combines shrimps, pasta, and various veggies for a burst of colors and flavors. A great pasta salad dish for lunch and guest food.

INGREDIENTS FOR 10 SERVINGS
- 12 oz. of three-colored penne pasta
- ½ pound of cooked shrimp
- ½ red bell pepper, diced
- ½ cup of red onion, chopped
- 3 stalks of celery
- 12 baby carrots, cut into thick slices
- 1 cup of cauliflower, cut into small round pieces
- ¼ cup of honey
- ¼ cup balsamic vinegar
- ½ tsp. of black pepper
- ½ tsp. garlic powder
- 1 tbsp. of French mustard
- ¾ cup of olive oil

METHOD
1. Cook pasta for around 10 minutes (or according to packaged instructions).
2. While pasta is boiling, cut all your veggies and place into a large mixing bowl. Add the cooked shrimp.
3. In a mixing bowl, add the honey, vinegar, black pepper, garlic powder, and mustard. While you whisk, slowly incorporate the oil and stir well.
4. Add in the drained pasta with the veggies and shrimp and gently combine everything together. Pour the liquid marinade over the pasta and veggies and toss to coat everything evenly.
5. Refrigerate for 3-5 hours prior to serving. Serve chilled.

NUTRITIONAL INFORMATION (Per Serving)

- Calories: 256kcal
- Carbohydrate: 41g
- Protein: 6.55g
- Sodium: 242.04mg
- Potassium: 131.88mg
- Phosphorus: 86.03mg
- Dietary Fiber: 2.28g
- Fat: 16.88g

Kidney Disease Stage 3

21. Steak and Onion Sandwich

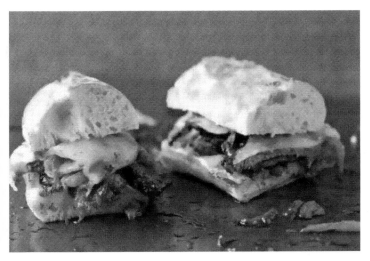

COOKING TIME: 8 MINUTES

DESCRIPTION

A rich steak sandwich that is very filling when you have to eat something good but don't have much time. Make this ahead for the next working day lunch or enjoy it fresh with the rest of your family.

INGREDIENTS FOR 4 SERVINGS

- 4 flank steaks (around 4 oz. each)
- 1 medium red onion, sliced
- 1 tbsp. of lemon juice
- 1 tbsp. of Italian seasoning
- 1 tsp. of black pepper
- 1 tbsp. of vegetable oil
- 4 sandwich/burger buns

METHOD

1. Wrap the steak with the lemon juice, the Italian seasoning, and pepper to taste. Cut into 4 pieces Heat the vegetable oil in a medium skillet over medium heat.
2. Cook steaks around 3 minutes on each side until you get a medium to well-done result. Take off and transfer onto a dish with absorbing paper.
3. In the same skillet, saute the onions until tender and transparent (around 3 minutes).
4. Cut the sandwich bun into half and place 1 piece of steak in each topped with the onions. Serve or wrap with paper or foil and keep in the fridge for the next day.

NUTRITIONAL INFORMATION (Per Serving)

- Calories: 315.26 kcal
- Carbohydrate: 8.47g
- Protein: 38.33g
- Sodium: 266.24mg
- Potassium: 238.2mg
- Phosphorus: 364.25mg
- Dietary Fiber: 0.76g
- Fat: 13.22g

Kidney Disease Stage 2

22. Zesty Crab Cakes

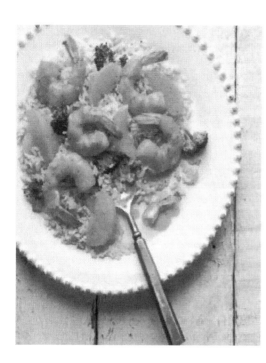

COOKING TIME: 6 MINUTES
DESCRIPTION
Crab cakes are a favorite dish in American seafood restaurants and are loved by kids and adults alike. If you like crab cakes, try this tasty recipe guilty-free as it is quite low on phosphorus and potassium.

INGREDIENTS FOR 6 SERVINGS
- 9 oz. (250 grams) of crab meat
- ⅓ cup of green or red bell pepper, thinly chopped
- ⅓ cup of low salt crackers, crushed
- ¼ cup of low-fat mayonnaise
- 1 tbsp. of dry mustard
- ½ tsp. of pepper
- 2 tbsp. of lemon juice
- ½ tsp. of lemon zest
- 1 tsp. of garlic powder
- 2 tbsp. of vegetable oil

METHOD
Mix all the ingredients except for the oil until uniform. Divide into 6 flat patties (around 5 inches in diameter).
Heat the vegetable oil in the skillet and shallow fry the patties for 2-3 minutes on each side (or until golden brown).
Serve warm on a dish with absorbing paper.

NUTRITIONAL INFORMATION (Per Serving)
- Calories: 144.42kcal
- Carbohydrate: 5.12g
- Protein: 8.47g
- Sodium: 212.31mg
- Potassium: 195mg
- Phosphorus: 127.42mg
- Dietary Fiber: 1.02g
- Fat: 9.2g

Kidney Disease Stage 5

23. Tofu Hoisin Sauté

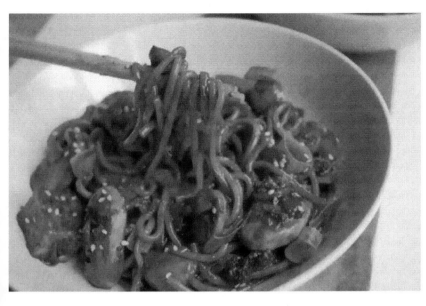

SERVES 4
PREP TIME: 15 MINUTES
COOK TIME: 20 MINUTES

If you are a fan of spicy, hot food, this will please your palate. A whole jalapeño pepper is used to create a complex heat that is not overwhelmingly mouth-scorching. If you want a relatively mild pepper, look for one that is green rather than red, and avoid peppers with white striations running lengthwise down the sides. These striations indicate that the pepper is older, which equates to infinitely hotter.

INGREDIENTS
- 2 tablespoons of hoisin sauce
- 2 tablespoons of rice vinegar
- 1 teaspoon of cornstarch
- 2 tablespoons of olive oil
- 1 (15-ounce) package extra-firm tofu, cut into 1-inch cubes
- 2 cups of unpeeled cubed eggplant
- 2 scallions, white and green parts, sliced
- 2 teaspoons of minced garlic
- 1 jalapeño pepper, minced
- 2 tablespoons of chopped fresh cilantro

METHOD
1. In a small bowl, whisk together the hoisin sauce, rice vinegar, and cornstarch and set aside.
2. In a large skillet over medium-high heat, heat the olive oil. Add the tofu, and sauté gently until golden brown, about 10 minutes, and transfer to a plate.
3. Reduce the heat to medium. Add the eggplant, scallions, garlic, and jalapeño pepper, and sauté until tender and fragrant, about 6 minutes.
4. Stir in the reserved sauce, and toss until the sauce thickens about 2

minutes. Stir in the tofu and cilantro, and serve hot.
5. Low-sodium tip Hoisin sauce is made with soy sauce, so it does contain a hefty amount of sodium per serving. This recipe would still be tasty, while slightly less intensely flavored if you use 1 tablespoon of hoisin sauce instead of 2 tablespoons.

NUTRITIONAL INFO
- PER SERVING Calories: 105
- Total fat: 4g
- Saturated fat: 1g
- Cholesterol: 0mg
- Sodium: 234mg
- Carbohydrates: 9g
- Fiber: 2g
- Phosphorus: 105mg
- Potassium: 192mg
- Protein: 8g

Kidney Disease Stage 2

24. Sweet Potato Curry

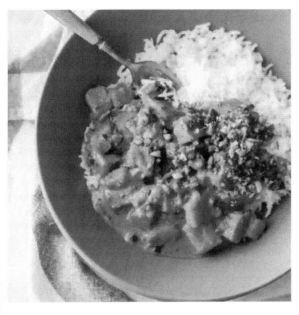

SERVES 6
PREP TIME: 20 MINUTES
COOK TIME: 20 MINUTES

LOW PROTEIN Sweet potatoes are relatively high in potassium, but the level is within range when consumed in a relatively small portion, like this curry. Sweet potatoes are an excellent source of beta-carotene, fiber, vitamin A, and vitamin C. Although you are probably used to vibrant orange sweet potatoes, don't be surprised if you ever cut into one and find deep purple flesh. Purple sweet potatoes contain anthocyanins, which are powerful antioxidants.

INGREDIENTS
- 2 teaspoons of olive oil
- 1 medium sweet onion, chopped
- 1 tablespoon of grated peeled fresh ginger
- 1 teaspoon of minced fresh garlic
- 2 cups of diced peeled sweet potatoes
- 1 cup of diced carrots
- 1 cup of water
- ½ cup of heavy (whipping) cream
- 1 tablespoon of curry powder
- 1 teaspoon of ground cumin
- 2 tablespoons of low-fat plain yogurt
- 2 tablespoons of chopped fresh cilantro

METHOD
1. In a large saucepan over medium-high heat, heat the olive oil.
2. Add the onion, ginger, and garlic and sauté until softened, about 3 minutes.

3. Add the sweet potatoes, carrots, water, cream, curry powder, and cumin and stir to mix well. Bring the mixture to a boil. Reduce the heat to low, and simmer until the vegetables are tender, about 15 minutes.
4. Serve immediately, topped with the yogurt and cilantro.

Substitution tip Almost any vegetable will work in a dish like curry, so let your creative impulses run wild. Stick to renal-friendly vegetables listed in this book (see Phosphorus, here, and Potassium, here) to ensure your mineral levels are within the correct range.

NUTRITIONAL INFO
- PER SERVING Calories: 132
- Total fat: 9g
- Saturated fat: 5g
- Cholesterol: 27mg
- Sodium: 40mg
- Carbohydrates: 13g
- Fiber: 2g
- Phosphorus: 48mg
- Potassium: 200mg
- Protein: 1g

Kidney Disease Stage 1

25. Zucchini Noodles With Spring Vegetables

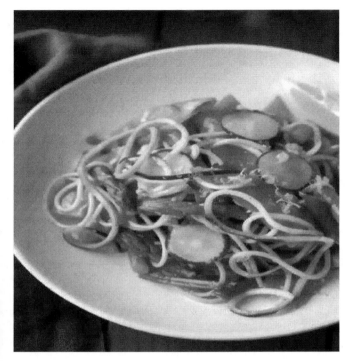

SERVES 6
PREP TIME: 20 MINUTES
COOK TIME: 10 MINUTES

LOW PROTEIN, LOW FAT Fresh and supremely inviting might describe the way heaps of vegetable noodles, asparagus spears, and plump cherry tomatoes look on your plate. Since they are vegetables, these noodles do not taste a thing like pasta, but you can still wind them around a fork and suck them up like spaghetti. If you get a medium to large, firm zucchini, and you have a spiralizer (see Cooking tip), you can spin out strands that are several feet in length, so you might want to snip them shorter—or not! (If you don't have a spiralizer, you can use a vegetable peeler to create the veggie noodles.) Zucchini noodles can keep in the refrigerator for up to 3 days in a sealed container.

INGREDIENTS
- 6 zucchini, cut into long noodles
- 1 cup of halved snow peas
- 1 cup (3-inch pieces) of asparagus
- 1 tablespoon of olive oil
- 1 teaspoon of minced fresh garlic
- 1 tablespoon of freshly squeezed lemon juice
- 1 cup of shredded fresh spinach
- ¾ cup of halved cherry tomatoes
- 2 tablespoons of chopped fresh basil leaves

METHOD
1. Fill a medium saucepan with water, place over medium-high heat, and bring to a boil.
2. Reduce the heat to medium, and blanch the zucchini ribbons, snow peas, and asparagus by submerging them in the water for 1 minute. Drain and rinse immediately under cold water.
3. Pat the vegetables dry with paper towels, and transfer to a large bowl.
4. Place a medium skillet over medium heat, and add the olive oil. Add the garlic, and sauté until tender, about 3 minutes.
5. Add the lemon juice and spinach, and sauté until the spinach is wilted about 3 minutes.
6. Add the zucchini mixture, the cherry tomatoes, and basil and toss until well combined.
7. Serve immediately.

Cooking tip: A spiralizer is a good investment. This inexpensive culinary tool can create the most delightful long noodles from fruit and vegetables for an inventive presentation.

NUTRITIONAL INFO
- PER SERVING Calories: 52
- Total fat: 2g
- Saturated fat: 0g
- Cholesterol: 0mg
- Sodium: 7mg
- Carbohydrates: 4g
- Fiber: 1g
- Phosphorus: 40mg
- Potassium: 197mg
- Protein: 2g

Kidney Disease Stage 4

26.   Stir-Fried Vegetables

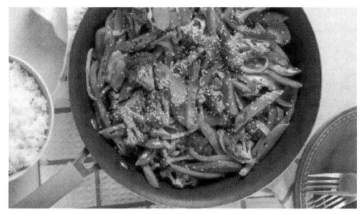

SERVES 4
PREP TIME: 15 MINUTES
COOK TIME: 15 MINUTES

LOW PROTEIN LOW FAT Broccoli is a base ingredient in many stir-fries because it cooks quickly and looks spectacular heaped with other vegetables with its tightly bunched florets. Broccoli is a cruciferous vegetable like cauliflower and cabbage, so it has the ability to lower cholesterol and detoxify the body. Broccoli can also help fight cancer. Be sure to not overcook this vegetable.

INGREDIENTS
- 2 teaspoons of olive oil
- ½ medium red onion, sliced
- 1 tablespoon of grated peeled fresh ginger
- 2 teaspoons of minced garlic
- 2 cups of broccoli florets
- 2 cups of cauliflower florets
- 1 red bell pepper, diced
- 1 cup of sliced carrots

METHOD
1. In a large skillet over medium-high heat, heat the olive oil.
2. Add the onion, ginger, and garlic and sauté until softened, about 3 minutes.
3. Add the broccoli, cauliflower, bell pepper, and carrots, and sauté until tender, about 10 minutes.
4. Serve hot.

Cooking tip: This dish is great served over steamed white basmati rice to create a satisfying meal. Avoid brown rice if you are watching your phosphorus levels because brown rice has twice as much phosphorus as white rice.

NUTRITIONAL INFO
- PER SERVING Calories: 50
- Total fat: 1g
- Saturated fat: 0g
- Cholesterol: 0mg
- Sodium: 26mg
- Carbohydrates: 6g
- Fiber: 2g
- Phosphorus: 36mg
- Potassium: 198mg
- Protein: 1g

Kidney Disease Stage 5

27. Lime Asparagus Spaghetti

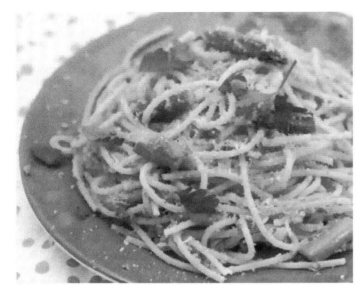

SERVES 6
PREP TIME: 5 MINUTES
COOK TIME: 20 MINUTES

LOW PROTEIN LOW FAT Asparagus has a fresh, almost grassy taste with a hint of sweetness, especially if you purchase the pencil-thin young asparagus. Part of the charm of this pretty salad is the long asparagus strips, which look like noodles. Asparagus is an excellent source of vitamin A, helping to support healthy eyes and reducing inflammation in the body.

INGREDIENTS

- 1 pound of asparagus spears, trimmed and cut into 2-inch pieces
- 2 teaspoons of olive oil
- 2 teaspoons of minced garlic
- 2 teaspoons of all-purpose flour
- 1 cup of Homemade Rice Milk (here, or use unsweetened store-bought) or almond milk
- Juice and zest of ½ lemon
- 1 tablespoon of chopped fresh thyme
- Freshly ground black pepper
- 2 cups of cooked spaghetti
- ¼ cup of grated Parmesan cheese

METHOD

1. Fill a large saucepan with water and bring to a boil over high heat. Add the asparagus and blanch until crisp-tender, about 2 minutes. Drain and set aside.
2. In a large skillet over medium-high heat, heat the olive oil. Add the garlic, and sauté until softened, about 2 minutes. Whisk in the flour to create a paste, about 1 minute. Whisk in the rice milk, lemon juice, lemon zest, and thyme.
3. Reduce the heat to medium and cook the sauce, whisking constantly, until thickened and creamy, about 3 minutes.

4. Season the sauce with pepper.
5. Stir in the spaghetti and the asparagus.
6. Serve the pasta topped with the Parmesan cheese.
7. Substitution tip Spaghetti looks lovely with the slender asparagus, but any pasta shape will work. Try farfalle, penne, or corkscrew cavatappi for this dish.

NUTRITIONAL INFO (per serving)
- Calories:127
- Total fat: 3g
- Saturated fat: 1g
- Cholesterol: 4mg
- Sodium: 67mg
- Carbohydrates: 19g
- Fiber: 2g
- Phosphorus 109mg
- Potassium: 200mg
- Protein: 6g

Kidney Disease Stage 2

28.   Garden Crustless Quiche

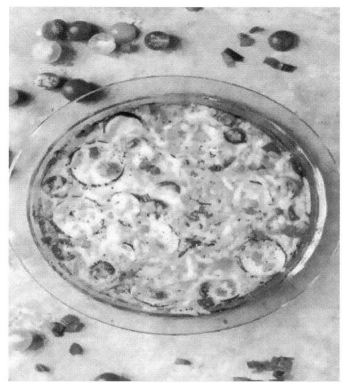

SERVES 6
PREP TIME: 10 MINUTES
COOK TIME: 25 MINUTES

Kale is the darling of today's nutrition world because it is packed with fiber, vitamins, and minerals. One cup of kale has over 1,000 percent of the daily recommended amount of vitamin K and 100 percent of the recommended vitamin A. Kale is lower in potassium than other dark leafy greens and it's high in iron, which is often deficient in those with kidney problems. Try different varieties of kale, because the taste and appearance of the various species can vary.

INGREDIENTS
- 6 eggs
- 2 egg whites
- ¼ cup of Homemade Rice Milk (here or use unsweetened store-bought)
- ¼ cup of shredded Swiss cheese, divided
- ¼ teaspoon of freshly ground black pepper
- 1 teaspoon of unsalted butter, plus more for the pie plate
- 1 teaspoon of minced garlic
- 1 scallion, white and green parts, chopped
- 1 yellow zucchini, chopped
- ½ cup of shredded stemmed kale
- 1 cup of quartered cherry tomatoes

METHOD

1. In a medium bowl, beat the eggs, egg whites, rice milk, half the swiss cheese, and the pepper until well blended, and set aside.
2. Preheat the oven to 350°F.
3. Grease a 9-inch pie plate with butter and set aside.
4. In a medium skillet over medium-high heat, melt 1 teaspoon of butter. Add the garlic and scallion, and sauté until softened, about 2 minutes.
5. Add the zucchini and kale, and sauté until wilted, about 3 minutes.
6. Transfer the vegetables from the skillet to the pie plate and add the tomatoes, spreading the vegetables evenly across the bottom.
7. Pour the egg mixture into the pie plate, and sprinkle with the remaining half of the Swiss cheese.
8. Bake until the quiche is puffed and lightly browned, 15 to 20 minutes.
9. Serve hot, warm, or cold.
10. Ingredient tip Yellow zucchini, sometimes called summer squash, is usually found lined up in a bin next to the more common green variety. You can interchange green with yellow in this dish.

NUTRITIONAL INFO

- PER SERVING Calories: 120
- Total fat: 8g
- Saturated fat: 4g
- Cholesterol: 221mg
- Sodium: 93mg
- Carbohydrates: 3g
- Fiber: 0g
- Phosphorus 120mg
- Potassium: 189mg
- Protein: 9g

Kidney Disease Stage 5

29. Lentil Veggie Burgers

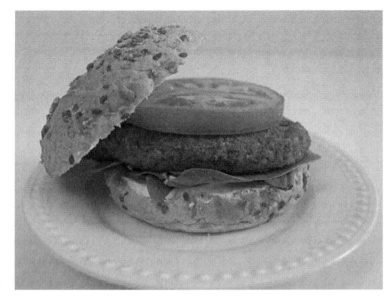

SERVES 4
PREP TIME: 15 MINUTES (PLUS 1 HOUR CHILLING TIME)
COOK TIME: 10 MINUTES

LOW FAT This underestimated familiar green is actually an incredible diuretic and very effective heavy metal detoxifier. Consuming parsley as part of your regular diet can reduce the risk of kidney stones and help treat existing urinary tract infections. Either flat-leaf or curly leaf parsley will do the trick because they taste almost the same and have an identical nutrition profile.

INGREDIENTS

- 2½ cups cooked white rice
- ½ cup cooked red lentils, drained and rinsed
- 2 eggs, lightly beaten
- 2 tablespoons chopped fresh parsley
- 2 teaspoons chopped fresh basil leaves
- Juice and zest of 1 lime
- 1 teaspoon minced garlic
- 1 tablespoon olive oil

METHOD

1. In a food processor (or blender), pulse the rice, lentils, eggs, parsley, basil, lime juice, lime zest, and garlic until the mixture holds together.
2. Transfer the rice mixture to a medium bowl, and set in the refrigerator until it firms up, about 1 hour.
3. Form the rice mixture into 4 patties.
4. In a large skillet over medium-high heat, heat the olive oil.

5. Add the veggie patties and cook until golden, about 5 minutes. Flip the patties over. Cook the other side for 5 minutes.
6. Transfer the burgers to a paper towel-lined plate.

Serve the veggie burgers hot with your favorite toppings.

NUTRITIONAL INFO
- Calories: 247
- Total fat: 7g
- Saturated fat: 2g
- Cholesterol: 106mg
- Sodium: 36mg
- Carbohydrates: 31g
- Fiber: 3g
- Phosphorus 120mg
- Potassium: 183mg
- Protein: 8g

Kidney Disease Stage 3

30. Baked Cauliflower Rice Cakes

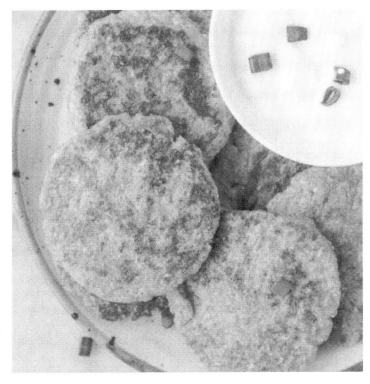

SERVES 6
PREP TIME: 10 MINUTES
COOK TIME: 20 MINUTES

A passerby might mistake these golden nuggets for unusual muffins because they are the same shape, but the savory cheesy taste of the rice cakes is unmistakable. From this recipe, one portion of the cooked rice, tender cauliflower, and creamy yogurt combination will fill you up easily, and is satisfying paired with a green salad

INGREDIENTS

- Olive oil for the pan
- 2 cups of chopped blanched cauliflower (see Cooking tip)
- 2 cups of cooked white basmati rice
- ¼ cup of plain yogurt
- 2 eggs, lightly beaten
- ½ cup of grated Cheddar cheese
- ¼ teaspoon of ground nutmeg
- Freshly ground black pepper

METHOD

1. Preheat the oven to 350°f.
2. Lightly coat 6 cups of a standard muffin tin with olive oil.
3. In a large bowl, mix together the cauliflower, rice, yogurt, eggs, cheese, and nutmeg.
4. Season the mixture with pepper.
5. Evenly divide the cauliflower mixture among the 6 prepared muffin cups.
6. Bake until golden and slightly puffy, about 20 minutes.
7. Let them stand for 5 minutes, then run a knife around the edges to loosen.
8. Serve hot, warm, or cold.

Cooking tip: To blanch the chopped cauliflower, plunge into boiling water for 3 minutes, then drain and rinse with cold water.

NUTRITIONAL INFO
- PER SERVING Calories: 141
- Total fat: 5g
- Saturated fat: 3g
- Cholesterol: 82mg
- Sodium: 98mg
- Carbohydrates: 18g
- Fiber: 1g
- Phosphorus 119mg
- Potassium: 178mg
- Protein: 7g

Kidney Disease Stage 5

Snacks Recipes

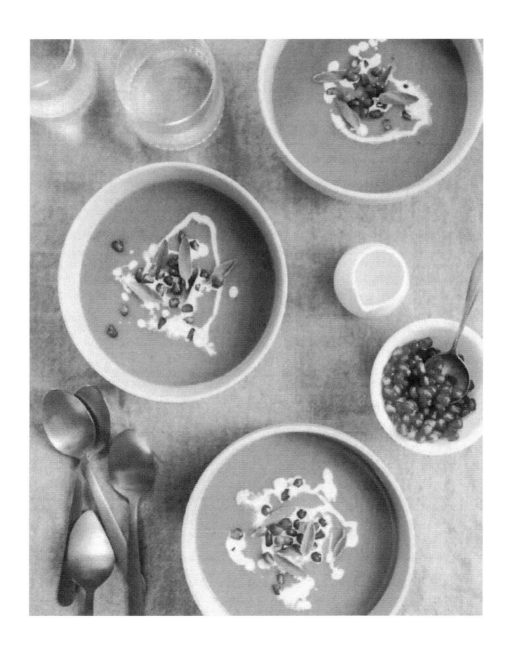

31. Cinnamon Apple Chips

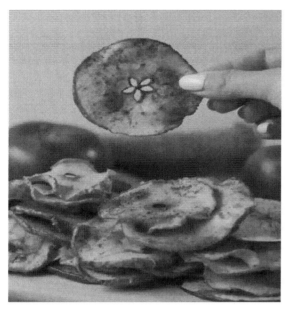

SERVES 4 • PREP TIME: 5 MINUTES
COOK TIME: 2 TO 3 HOURS

There's something about crunchy snacks like chips that leave you reaching for more. This guilt-free chip provides vitamins, fiber, and delicious flavor all in one. Cinnamon, an aromatic and warming spice, aids in digestion and supports the spleen, kidneys, and lungs, making it a great addition to your diet and to these chips.

INGREDIENTS

- 4 apples
- 1 teaspoon ground cinnamon

METHOD

1. Preheat the oven to 200°F. Line a baking sheet with parchment paper.
2. Core the apples and cut into ⅛-inch slices.
3. In a medium bowl, toss the apple slices with the cinnamon. Spread the apples in a single layer on the prepared baking sheet.
4. Cook for 2 to 3 hours, until the apples are dry. They will still be soft while hot but will crisp once completely cooled. Store in an airtight container for up to four days.

Cooking tip: If you don't have parchment paper, use cooking spray to prevent sticking.

NUTRITIONAL INFO

- Per serving Calories: 96
- Total fat: 0g
- Saturated fat: 0g
- Cholesterol: 0mg
- Sodium: 2mg
- Carbohydrates: 26g
- Fiber: 5g
- Phosphorus 0mg
- Potassium: 198mg
- Protein: 1g

Kidney Disease Stage 2

32. Savory Collard Chips

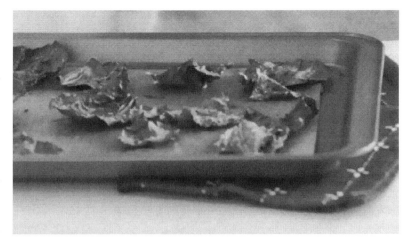

SERVES 4 • PREP TIME: 5 MINUTES
COOK TIME: 20 MINUTES

If you like kale chips, you'll probably love collard chips. The sturdy green holds up well to baking, creating a crisp chip that is perfect for any time snacking. The simple mix of herbs adds a garlicky kick to the chips, which will ensure that you are getting plenty of vegetables in your diet—even if they don't feel like vegetables.

INGREDIENTS

- 1 bunch of collard greens
- 1 teaspoon of extra-virgin olive oil
- Juice of ½ lemon
- ½ teaspoon of garlic powder
- ¼ teaspoon of freshly ground black pepper

METHOD

1. Preheat the oven to 350°F. Line a baking sheet with parchment paper.
2. Cut the collards into 2-by-2-inch squares and pat dry with paper towels. In a large bowl, toss the greens with the olive oil, lemon juice, garlic powder, and pepper. Use your hands to mix well, massaging the dressing into the greens until evenly coated.
3. Arrange the collards in a single layer on the baking sheet, and cook for 8 minutes. Flip the pieces and cook for an additional 8 minutes, until crisp. Remove from the oven, let cool, and store in an airtight container in a cool location for up to three days.

Substitution tip: If you prefer, use fresh garlic instead of dried. Mince 2 or 3 cloves, toss with the collards and proceed as directed.

NUTRITIONAL INFO

- Calories: 24
- Total fat: 1g
- Saturated fat: 0g
- Cholesterol: 0mg

- Sodium: 8mg
- Carbohydrates: 3g
- Fiber: 1g
- Phosphorus 6mg
- Potassium: 72mg
- Protein: 1g

Kidney Disease Stage 1

33. Roasted Red Pepper Hummus

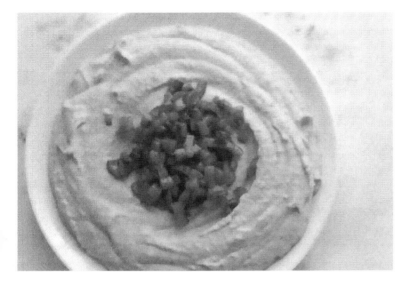

SERVES 8 • PREP TIME: 10 MINUTES
COOK TIME: 10 MINUTES

Hummus is generally considered a healthy food, but like many other processed foods, store-bought versions are filled with sodium and preservatives. Make this simple hummus at home to keep sodium levels in check, and keep the serving size to 2 tablespoons. This is easy if you use it as a spread on sandwiches, or make vegetables the star and dip them in hummus for a quick snack.

INGREDIENTS

- 1 red bell pepper
- 1 (15-ounce) can chickpeas, drained and rinsed
- Juice of 1 lemon
- 2 tablespoons of tahini
- 2 garlic cloves
- 2 tablespoons of extra-virgin olive oil

METHOD

1. Move an oven rack to the highest position. Heat the broiler to high.
2. Core the pepper and cut it into three or four large pieces. Arrange them on a baking sheet, skin-side up.
3. Broil the peppers for 5 to 10 minutes, until the skins are charred. Remove from the oven and transfer the peppers to a small bowl. Cover with plastic wrap and let them steam for 10 to 15 minutes, until cool enough to handle.
4. Peel the charred skin off the peppers, and place the peppers in a blender.
5. Add the chickpeas, lemon juice, tahini, garlic, and olive oil. Process until smooth, adding up to 1 tablespoon of water to adjust consistency as desired.

Substitution tip: This hummus can also be made without the red pepper if desired. To do this, simply follow Step 5. This will cut the potassium to 59mg per serving.

NUTRITIONAL INFO
- Per serving Calories: 103
- Total fat: 6g
- Saturated fat: 1g
- Cholesterol: 0mg
- Carbohydrates: 10g
- Fiber: 3g
- Protein: 3g
- Phosphorus 58mg
- Potassium: 91mg
- Sodium: 72mg

Kidney Disease Stage 2

34. Thai-Style Eggplant Dip

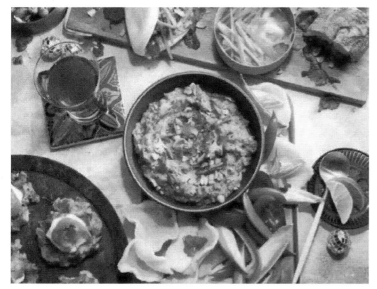

SERVES 4 • PREP TIME: 10 MINUTES
COOK TIME: 30 MINUTES

In hot climates, such as Thailand, eggplant is commonplace as a cooling vegetable with its sweet flavor. Here it's mixed with sweet, savory, and spicy elements to create a fantastic dip that is just right for vegetables or crackers.

INGREDIENTS

- 1-pound of Thai eggplant (or Japanese or Chinese eggplant)
- 2 tablespoons of rice vinegar
- 2 teaspoons of sugar
- 1 teaspoon of low-sodium soy sauce
- 1 jalapeño pepper
- 2 garlic cloves
- ¼ cup of chopped basil
- Cut vegetables or crackers, for serving

METHOD

1. Preheat the oven to 425°F.
2. Pierce the eggplant in several places with a skewer or knife. Place on a rimmed baking sheet and cook until soft, about 30 minutes. Let cool, cut in half, and scoop out the flesh of the eggplant into a blender.
3. Add the rice vinegar, sugar, soy sauce, jalapeño, garlic, and basil to the blender. Process until smooth. Serve with cut vegetables or crackers.
4. Lower sodium tip: If you need to lower your sodium further, omit the soy sauce to lower the sodium to 3mg.

NUTRITIONAL INFO

- Calories: 40
- Total fat: 0g
- Saturated fat: 0g
- Cholesterol: 0mg
- Carbohydrates: 10g
- Fiber: 4g

- Protein: 2g
- Phosphorus 34mg
- Potassium: 284mg

Kidney Disease Stage 3

35.   Collard Salad Rolls with Peanut Dipping Sauce

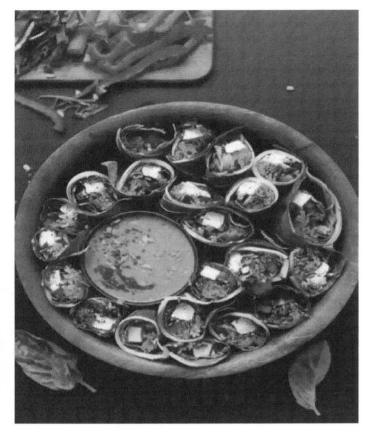

SERVES 4 • PREP TIME: 20 MINUTES

These delicious Asian-inspired rolls allow you to creatively load up on vegetables. Perfect as a midday snack or light lunch, the rolls possess a wonderful variety of textures and flavor, and when dunked in the sweet-and-spicy peanut-butter dipping sauce, they'll reward you with an explosion of taste.

INGREDIENTS

FOR THE DIPPING SAUCE
- ¼ cup of peanut butter
- 2 tablespoons of honey
- Juice of 1 lime
- ¼ teaspoon of red chili flakes

FOR THE SALAD ROLLS
- 4 ounces of extra-firm tofu
- 1 bunch of collard greens
- 1 cup of thinly sliced purple cabbage
- 1 cup of bean sprouts
- 2 carrots, cut into matchsticks
- ½ cup of cilantro leaves and stems

METHOD
1. TO MAKE THE DIPPING SAUCE
2. In a blender, combine the peanut butter, honey, lime juice, and chili flakes, and process until smooth. Add 1 to 2 tablespoons of water as desired for consistency.
3. TO MAKE THE SALAD ROLLS
4. Using paper towels, press the excess moisture from the tofu. Cut into ½-inch-thick matchsticks.
5. Remove any tough stems from the collard greens and set aside.
6. Arrange all of the ingredients within reach. Cup one collard green leaf in your hand, and add a couple of pieces of the tofu and a small amount each of the cabbage, bean sprouts, and

carrots. Top with a couple of cilantro sprigs, and roll into a cylinder. Place each roll, seam-side down, on a serving platter while you assemble the rest of the rolls. Serve with the dipping sauce.

Substitution tip: To lower the potassium, omit the cabbage and use only 1 carrot, which will drop the potassium to 208mg.

NUTRITIONAL INFO
- Calories: 174
- Total fat: 9g
- Saturated fat: 2g
- Cholesterol: 0mg
- Carbohydrates: 20g
- Fiber: 5g
- Protein: 8g
- Phosphorus 56mg
- Potassium: 284mg
- Sodium: 42mg

Kidney Disease Stage 2

36. Roasted Mint Carrots

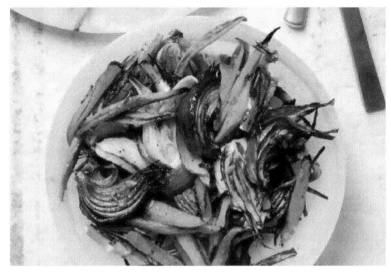

SERVES 6 • PREP TIME: 5 MINUTES
COOK TIME: 20 MINUTES

Carrots are a great source of the antioxidant vitamin A, and although high in potassium, consumed in moderation carrots can be a healthy part of your diet. In this preparation, roasting enhances the vegetable's natural sweetness while mint adds a complementary flavor. There are several hundred varieties of carrots, but seek out those with the deepest orange color, as they contain the most vitamin A.

INGREDIENTS
- 1 pound of carrots, trimmed
- 1 tablespoon of extra-virgin olive oil
- Freshly ground black pepper
- ¼ cup of thinly sliced mint

METHOD
1. Preheat the oven to 425°F.
2. Arrange the carrots in a single layer on a rimmed baking sheet. Drizzle with the olive oil, and shake the carrots on the sheet to coat. Season with pepper.
3. Roast for 20 minutes, or until tender and browned, stirring twice while cooking. Sprinkle with the mint and serve.

Substitution tip: To lower the potassium in this dish, use 8 ounces of carrots and 8 ounces of turnips cut into cubes. This will cut the potassium to 193mg.

NUTRITIONAL INFO
- Per serving Calories: 51
- Total fat: 2g
- Saturated fat: 4g
- Cholesterol: 0mg
- Carbohydrates: 7g
- Fiber: 2g

- Protein: 1g
- Phosphorus 26mg
- Potassium: 242mg
- Sodium: 52mg

Kidney Disease Stage 4

37. Roasted Root Vegetables

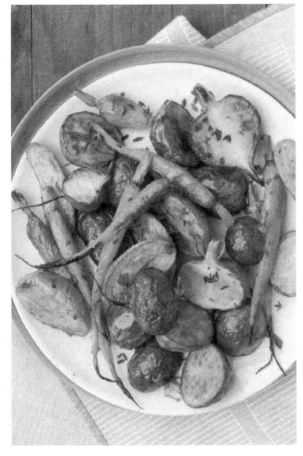

SERVES 6 • PREP TIME: 10 MINUTES
COOK TIME: 25 MINUTES

Root vegetables have a comfort-food appeal that makes them great for pairing with, fish, and poultry dishes. Turnips, rutabaga, and parsnips may not be the first root vegetables you think of, but these nutritional powerhouses are well worth experimenting with. Roasting accentuates their sweetness, resulting in a tender mix that's loaded with flavor but doesn't overwhelm the main course. Look for young and tender vegetables—you don't need to peel them, so prep time is short.

INGREDIENTS

- 1 cup of chopped turnips
- 1 cup of chopped rutabaga
- 1 cup of chopped parsnips
- 1 tablespoon of extra-virgin olive oil
- 1 teaspoon of fresh chopped rosemary
- Freshly ground black pepper

METHOD

1. Preheat the oven to 400°F.
2. In a large bowl, toss the turnips, rutabaga, and parsnips with the olive oil and rosemary. Arrange in a single layer on a baking sheet, and season with pepper.
3. Bake until the vegetables are tender and browned, 20 to 25 minutes, stirring once.

Substitution tip: Experiment with other fresh herbs in this dish to suit your own tastes. Thyme, tarragon, oregano, and minced garlic all add unique flavors to these root vegetables.

NUTRITIONAL INFO

- Per serving Calories: 52
- Total fat: 2g
- Saturated fat: 0g
- Cholesterol: 0mg

- Carbohydrates: 7g
- Fiber: 2g
- Protein: 1g
- Phosphorus 35mg
- Potassium: 205mg
- Sodium: 22mg

Kidney Disease Stage 3

38. Vegetable Couscous

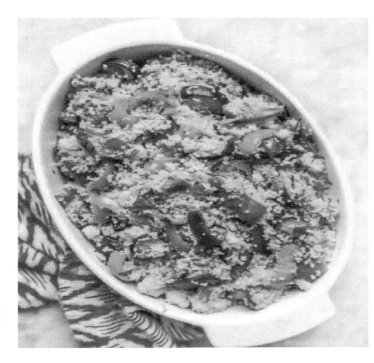

SERVES 6 • PREP TIME: 10 MINUTES
COOK TIME: 15 MINUTES

Couscous is a quick-cooking refined grain product, great for weeknight meals. Simply add to boiling water, cover, let stand for just under 10 minutes, and voilà—this delicious grain is ready! Combined with vegetables, this filling side dish pairs well with, seafood, and chicken.

INGREDIENTS

- 1 tablespoon of extra-virgin olive oil
- ½ sweet onion, diced
- 1 carrot, diced
- 1 celery stalk, diced
- ½ cup of diced red or yellow bell pepper
- 1 small zucchini, diced
- 1 cup of couscous
- 1½ cups of Simple Chicken Broth or low-sodium store-bought chicken stock
- ½ teaspoon of garlic powder
- Freshly ground black pepper

METHOD

1. In a large skillet, heat the olive oil over medium heat. Add the onion, carrot, celery, and bell pepper, and cook, stirring occasionally.
2. Add the zucchini, couscous, broth, and garlic powder. Stir to blend, and bring to a boil. Cover and remove from the heat. Let stand for 5 to 8 minutes. Fluff with a fork, season with pepper and serve.

Substitution tip: Swap out vegetables to make this couscous your own creation. Yellow summer squash or pattypan squash can be substituted for the zucchini. Other vegetables, like asparagus, broccoli, or cauliflower, can be added instead of carrots and bell peppers.

NUTRITIONAL INFO

- Per serving Calories: 154
- Total fat: 3g

- Saturated fat: 1g
- Cholesterol: 0mg
- Carbohydrates: 27g
- Fiber: 2g
- Protein: 5g
- Phosphorus 83mg
- Potassium: 197mg
- Sodium: 36mg

Kidney Disease Stage 2

39. Garlic Cauliflower Rice

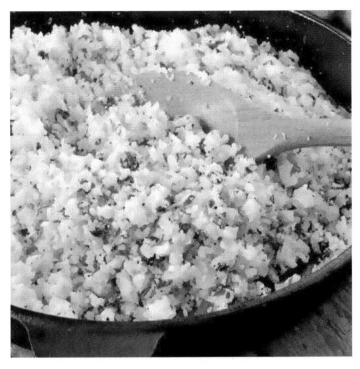

**SERVES 8 • PREP TIME: 5 MINUTES
COOK TIME: 10 MINUTES**

Cauliflower rice is a clever vegetable-based alternative to white or brown rice. In this version, garlic and freshly ground black pepper make for a flavorful blend that goes well with vegetarian dishes. Because cauliflower is high in potassium, I recommend keeping the serving size at just ½ cup.

INGREDIENTS
- 1 medium head cauliflower
- 1 tablespoon of extra-virgin olive oil
- 4 garlic cloves, minced
- Freshly ground black pepper

METHOD
1. Using a sharp knife, remove the core of the cauliflower, and separate the cauliflower into florets.
2. In a food processor, pulse the florets until they are the size of rice, being careful not to over-process them to the point of becoming mushy.
3. In a large skillet over medium heat, heat the olive oil. Add the garlic, and stir until just fragrant.
4. Add the cauliflower, stirring to coat. Add 1 tablespoon of water to the pan, cover, and reduce the heat to low. Steam for 7 to 10 minutes, until the cauliflower is tender. Season with pepper and serve.

Cooking tip: Cauliflower rice tastes great both when fresh and after resting in the refrigerator for a day or two. Make a batch and use it throughout the week as a side dish, heating it in the microwave before serving. In an airtight container, it will keep refrigerated for three to five days.

NUTRITIONAL INFO
- Per serving Calories: 37
- Total fat: 2g

- Saturated fat: 0g
- Cholesterol: 0mg
- Carbohydrates: 4g
- Fiber: 2g
- Protein: 2g
- Phosphorus 35mg
- Potassium: 226mg
- Sodium: 22mg

Kidney Disease Stage 4

40. Celery and Arugula Salad

SERVES 4 • PREP TIME: 10 MINUTES

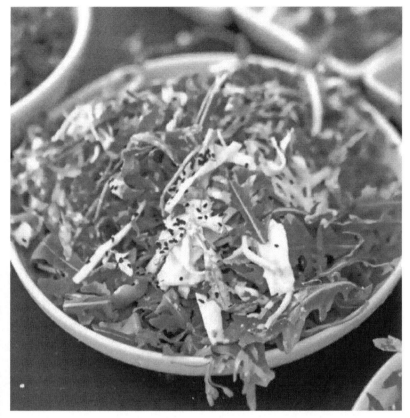

Peppery arugula makes a wonderful complement to the crunch of celery in this salad. Arugula is a bitter digestive aide and a terrific source of vitamins A and C, calcium, and folic acid. Find it in markets in the spring, early summer, and fall, or try your hand at growing your own. Arugula is easy to grow from seeds and will provide you with plenty of salads in no time.

INGREDIENTS

- 1 shallot, thinly sliced
- 3 celery stalks, cut into 1-inch pieces about ¼ inch thick
- 2 cups of loosely packed arugula
- 1 tablespoon of extra-virgin olive oil
- 2 tablespoons of white wine vinegar
- Freshly ground black pepper
- 2 tablespoons of grated Parmesan cheese

METHOD

1. In a medium bowl, toss the shallot, celery stalks, and arugula.
2. In a small bowl, whisk the olive oil, vinegar, and pepper. Pour the dressing over the salad, and toss to coat. Top with Parmesan cheese and serve.

Substitution tip: For a milder salad, you can substitute an equal amount of baby salad greens, or mix 1 cup of salad greens and 1 cup of arugula.

NUTRITIONAL INFO
- Per serving Calories: 45
- Total fat: 4g
- Saturated fat: 1g
- Cholesterol: 2mg
- Carbohydrates: 1g
- Fiber: 0g
- Protein: 1g
- Phosphorus 23mg
- Potassium: 47mg
- Sodium: 47mg

Kidney Disease Stage 5

41. Cucumber and Radish Salad

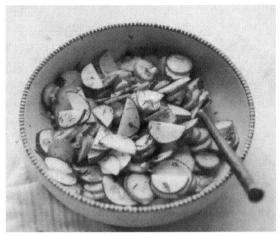

SERVES 6 •
PREP TIME: 10 MINUTES

If you love the snap of cucumbers and radishes, this salad will please your palate. Both vegetables are sources of potassium, however, so it's important to keep the serving size to ½ cup. For the best flavor and nutrition, use raw apple cider vinegar, characterized by cloudy sediment at the bottom of the bottle.

INGREDIENTS

- 2 large cucumbers, peeled and sliced
- 1 bunch of radishes, sliced
- ½ sweet onion, sliced
- ¼ cup of apple cider vinegar
- 1 tablespoon of extra-virgin olive oil
- Freshly ground black pepper

METHOD

1. In a medium bowl, toss the cucumbers, radishes, and onion.
2. Add the apple cider vinegar and olive oil, and toss to coat. Season with pepper.

Cooking tip: Make this salad up to two days in advance and store refrigerated in an airtight container until ready for use.

NUTRITIONAL INFO

- Per serving Calories: 69
- Total fat: 8g
- Saturated fat: 1g
- Cholesterol: 0mg
- Carbohydrates: 8g
- Fiber: 2g
- Protein: 2g
- Phosphorus 52mg
- Potassium: 386mg
- Sodium: 29mg

Kidney Disease Stage 4

42.   Spinach Salad with Orange Vinaigrette

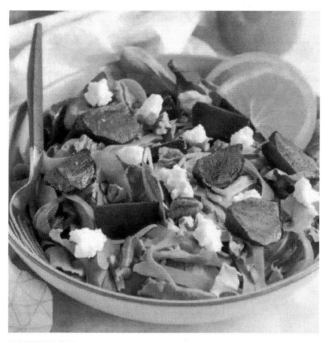

SERVES 4 •
PREP TIME: 5 MINUTES

This super-quick, refreshing salad presents itself with a touch of sweetness and a treasure trove of nutrients. Vitamins A, C, K, and fiber are just a few of its hidden health benefits. To ensure that the greens stay crispy, toss the salad with the vinaigrette right before serving.

INGREDIENTS

- Zest and juice of 1 mandarin orange
- 1 tablespoon of extra-virgin olive oil
- Freshly ground black pepper
- 6 ounces baby spinach
- 2 mandarin oranges, peeled, membranes removed

METHOD

1. In a small bowl, whisk the orange zest, orange juice, and olive oil. Season with pepper.
2. In a medium bowl, toss the spinach and pieces of orange. Drizzle the dressing over the salad, and toss to coat. Serve.

Substitution tip: To make a heartier and stand-alone salad as a meal, add 1 cup of diced avocado. This will increase the fat content to 9g, the phosphorus to 53mg, and the potassium to 535mg.

NUTRITIONAL INFO

- Per serving Calories: 73
- Total fat: 4g
- Saturated fat: 1g
- Cholesterol: 0mg
- Carbohydrates: 10g
- Fiber: 2g
- Protein: 2g
- Phosphorus 33mg
- Potassium: 353mg
- Sodium: 35mg

Kidney Disease Stage 3

43. Mixed Green Leaf and Citrus Salad

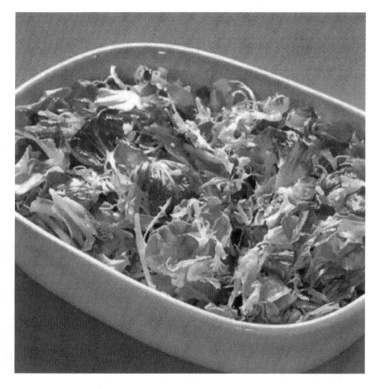

SERVES 4 • PREP TIME: 10 MINUTES

This sweet and savory combination of citrus, olives, and cranberries is nothing short of addictive. Pepitas, which are hulled pumpkin seeds of a South and Central American variety of squash, contain more protein than many other nuts and seeds, plus they provide the salad with a great crunch. Used sparingly here because of that protein, the pepitas combine with cranberries and olives to create a fun mix of textures and flavors.

INGREDIENTS

- 4 cups of mixed salad greens
- ¼ cup of pepitas
- Juice of 1 lemon
- 2 teaspoons of extra-virgin olive oil
- Freshly ground black pepper
- 1 orange, peeled and thinly sliced
- ½ lemon, peeled and thinly sliced
- 4 tablespoons of (¼cup) dried cranberries
- 4 tablespoons of (¼cup) pitted Kalamata olives

METHOD

1. In a large bowl, toss the greens, pepitas, lemon juice, and olive oil. Season with pepper.
2. Arrange the greens on four plates, and top each with 2 slices of orange and lemon. Add 1 tablespoon each of cranberries and Kalamata olives to each plate. Serve.
3. Ingredient tip: Toasted pepitas are delicious in this salad. To toast them, preheat the oven to 25°F. Toss the pepitas with ½ teaspoon of olive oil, then spread them on a baking sheet. Roast for about 15 minutes, until golden. Let cool before adding to the salad.

Substitution tip: Use any combination of citrus in this salad for different effects. Sliced grapefruit, limes, and different types of oranges can all be used based on your preference.

NUTRITIONAL INFO
- Per serving Calories: 142
- Total fat: 9g
- Saturated fat: 1g
- Cholesterol: 0mg
- Carbohydrates: 15g
- Fiber: 2g
- Protein: 3g
- Phosphorus 116mg
- Potassium: 219mg
- Sodium: 137mg

Kidney Disease Stage 4

44. Roasted Beet Salad

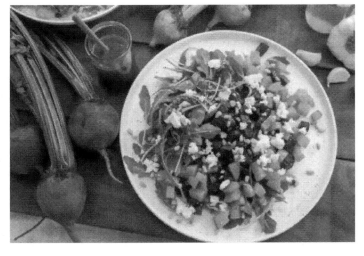

SERVES 4 • PREP TIME: 10 MINUTES
COOK TIME: 30 MINUTES

Roasting vegetables transforms them into sweet morsels, and considering how sweet the beet starts off, its flavor is all the more pronounced when roasted. For a light meal, serve this decadent salad topped with feta and walnuts, or pair it with a poultry dish for something heartier. Select small beets when making this salad—they cook quicker and make for a lovely presentation on the plate.

INGREDIENTS
- 8 small beets, trimmed
- 2 tablespoons of plus 1 teaspoon extra-virgin olive oil, divided
- 1 tablespoon of white wine vinegar
- 1 teaspoon of Dijon mustard
- Freshly ground black pepper
- 4 cups of baby salad greens
- ½ sweet onion, sliced
- 2 tablespoons of crumbled feta cheese
- 2 tablespoons of walnut pieces

METHOD
1. Preheat the oven to 400°F.
2. Toss the beets with 1 teaspoon of olive oil, wrap them in aluminum foil, and cook for 30 minutes, until fork-tender.
3. In a small bowl, whisk the remaining 2 tablespoons of olive oil, vinegar, and mustard. Season with pepper.
4. In a medium bowl, mix the salad greens, onion, feta cheese, and walnuts. Toss with about half of the vinaigrette. Arrange on four plates.
5. Slice the beets into wedges and top the salads. Serve with the remaining dressing.

Cooking tip: To make this salad in advance, just assemble the salad greens, onion, feta, and walnuts in a bowl—hold off on tossing it with the vinaigrette until ready to serve, to prevent wilting. Store refrigerated up to three days before serving.

NUTRITIONAL INFO
- Per serving Calories: 170
- Total fat: 9g
- Saturated fat: 2g
- Cholesterol: 4mg
- Carbohydrates: 20g
- Fiber: 5g
- Protein: 4g
- Phosphorus 93mg
- Potassium: 585mg
- Sodium: 217mg

Kidney Disease Stage 3

45. Pear and Watercress Salad

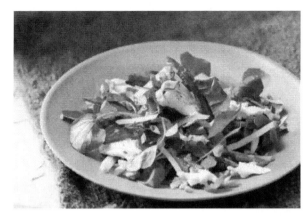

SERVES 4 • PREP TIME: 10 MINUTES

A pungent herb with a mustard-like flavor, watercress feels surprisingly cool in the mouth. Mixed with pear, this refreshing fall salad simply pops with flavor. For best results, use pears that hold their shapes, such as Seckel, Comice, or Bosc.

INGREDIENTS

- ¼ cup of sweet onion, coarsely chopped
- 1 teaspoon of Dijon mustard
- 2 tablespoons of extra-virgin olive oil
- 1 tablespoon of white wine vinegar
- 1 teaspoon of honey
- 1 bunch watercress, thick stems removed, washed well
- 2 ripe pears, cored and cut into wedges
- 1 ounce of crumbled feta cheese

METHOD

1. In a food processor or blender, combine the onion, mustard, olive oil, vinegar, and honey. Process until smooth.
2. In a medium bowl, toss the watercress with the dressing. Arrange on four plates. Top each with pear slices and crumbled feta cheese.
3. Ingredient tip: Watercress is extremely perishable, so you'll want to buy it within a day or two of using it. To store it, place the stems in water without immersing the leaves. When ready to use, wash the leaves in a bowl of water, changing the water out several times before draining and using.

NUTRITIONAL INFO

- Per serving Calories: 120
- Total fat: 8g
- Saturated fat: 4g
- Cholesterol: 221mg
- Carbohydrates: 3g
- Fiber: 0g

- Protein: 9g
- Phosphorus 120mg
- Potassium: 189mg
- Sodium: 93mg

Kidney Disease Stage 4

Dinner Recipes

1. **Vegetable Lover's Chicken Soup**

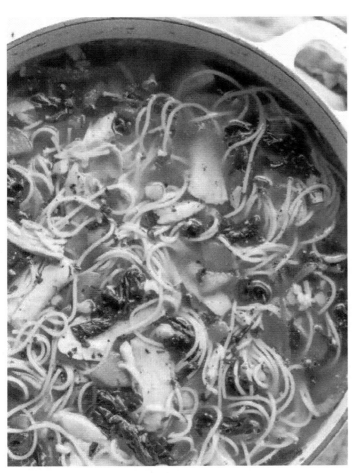

SERVES: 6
COOKING TIME: 20 MINUTES

INGREDIENTS:
- 1 ½ cups of baby spinach
- 2 tbsp. of orzo (tiny pasta)
- 1 tbsp. of dry white wine
- 1 14oz of low sodium chicken broth
- 2 plum tomatoes, chopped
- ½ tsp. of Italian seasoning
- 1 large shallot, chopped
- 1 small zucchini, diced
- 8oz of chicken tenders
- 1 tbsp. of extra virgin olive oil

METHOD
1. In a large saucepan, heat oil over medium heat and add the chicken. Stir occasionally for four minutes until browned. Transfer on a plate. Set aside.
2. In the same saucepan, add the zucchini, Italian seasoning, shallot, and salt and stir often until the vegetables are softened.
3. Add the tomatoes, wine, broth, and orzo and increase the heat to high to bring the mixture to boil. Reduce the heat and simmer for 3 minutes.
4. Add the cooked chicken and stir in the spinach last.
5. Serve hot.

NUTRITION INFORMATION:
- Per serving Calories: 80
- Carbohydrates: 5g
- Protein: 10g
- Fats: 3g
- Phosphorus 112mg
- Potassium: 258mg
- Sodium: 75mg

Kidney Disease Stage 2

46. Creamy Pumpkin Soup

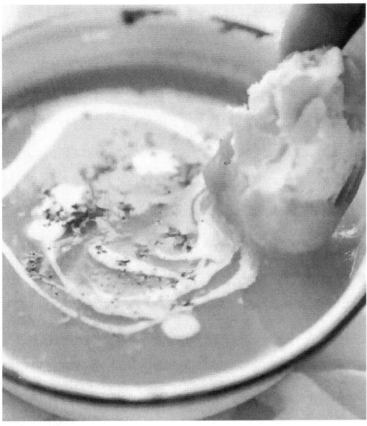

SERVES: 4
COOKING TIME: 20 MINUTES

INGREDIENTS:
- 1 onion, chopped
- 1 slice of bacon
- 2 tsp. of ground ginger
- 1 tsp. of cinnamon
- 1 cup of applesauce
- 3 ½ cups of low sodium chicken broth
- 1 29-oz can pumpkin
- Pepper to taste
- ½ cup of light sour cream

METHOD
1. On medium-high fire, place a soup pot and add bacon once hot. Sauté until crispy, around 5 minutes.
2. Discard bacon fat, before continuing to cook.
3. Add ginger, applesauce, chicken broth, and pumpkin. Lightly season with pepper.
4. Bring to a simmer and cook for 10 minutes.
5. Taste and adjust seasoning.
6. Turn off fire, stir in sour cream and mix well.
7. Serve and enjoy while hot.

NUTRITION INFORMATION:
- Per serving Calories: 224
- Carbohydrates: 34g
- Protein: 8g
- Fats: 8g

- Phosphorus: 188mg
- Potassium: 855mg
- Sodium: 132mg

Kidney Disease Stage 4

47. Broccoli, Arugula and Avocado Cream Soup

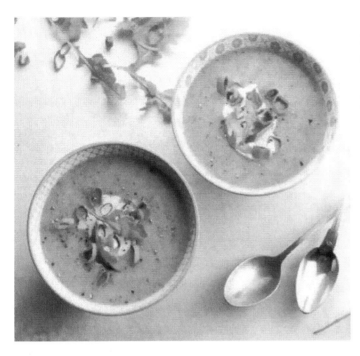

SERVES: 2
COOKING TIME: 10 MINUTES

INGREDIENTS:
- ¼ tsp. of red pepper flakes
- ½ Haas avocado
- 1 cup of water
- 1 tbsp. of apple cider vinegar
- 1 tbsp. of honey
- 1 tbsp. of olive oil
- 1/3 medium onion
- 1-inch minced ginger root
- 2 handfuls arugula
- 8-10 decent sized broccoli clusters
- Juice from half a lemon

METHOD
1. Steam broccoli for at least 5-7 minutes or until bright green.
2. In a saucepan, on medium-high fire and heat oil. Add onions and sauté until translucent.
3. In a blender, add all ingredients including cooked onion and broccoli plus a half cup of water.
4. Blend until smooth and creamy.
5. You can serve hot or cold.

NUTRITION INFORMATION:
- Calories per Serving: 206
- Carbs: 20g
- Protein: 3g fats: 14g
- Phosphorus: 75mg
- Potassium: 529mg
- Sodium: 25mg
- Kidney Disease Stage 2

Kidney Disease Stage 2

48. Salad Greens with Roasted Beets

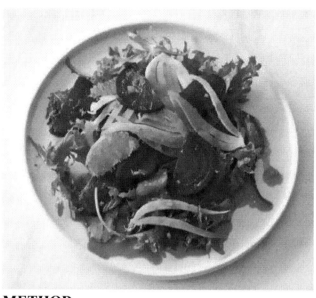

SERVES: 4
COOKING TIME: 60 MINUTES

INGREDIENTS:
- ¼ cup of extra-virgin olive oil
- ½ cup of chopped walnuts
- ½ teaspoon of Dijon mustard
- 1 tablespoon of dried cranberries, chopped roughly
- 1 tablespoon of minced red onions
- 2 tablespoons of sherry vinegar
- 3 medium beets, washed and trimmed
- 4 cups of baby spinach

METHOD
1. In foil, wrap beets and bake in a preheated 400oF oven. Bake until beets are tender, around 1 hour. Once done, open foil and allow it to cool. When cool to touch, peel beets and dice.
2. Mix well mustard, red onions, vinegar, and olive oil. Mix in spinach, beets, and cranberries. Toss to coat well.

NUTRITION INFORMATION:
- Calories per Serving: 190
- Carbohydrates: 11g
- Protein: 4g
- Fats: 16g
- Phosphorus: 94mg
- Potassium: 447mg
- Sodium: 195mg

Kidney Disease Stage 1

49. Nutty and Fruity Garden Salad

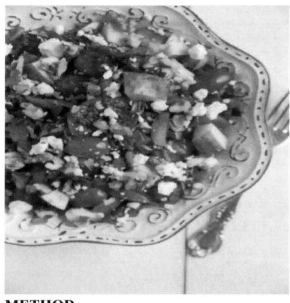

SERVES: 3
COOKING TIME: 0 MINUTES

INGREDIENTS:
- ½ cup of chopped walnuts, toasted
- 1 ripe persimmon, sliced
- 1 ripe red pear, sliced
- 1 shallot, minced
- 1 teaspoon of garlic minced
- 1 teaspoon of wholegrain mustard
- 2 tablespoons of fresh lemon juice
- 3 tablespoons of extra virgin olive oil
- 6 cups of baby spinach

METHOD
1. Mix well garlic, shallot, oil, lemon juice, and mustard in a large salad bowl.
2. Add spinach, pear, and persimmon. Toss to coat well.
3. To serve, garnish with chopped pecans.

NUTRITION INFORMATION:
- Calories: per Serving: 277
- Carbohydrates: 25g
- Protein: 6g
- Fats: 19g
- Phosphorus: 125mg
- Potassium: 610mg
- Sodium: 170mg

Kidney Disease Stage 2

50.   Roasted Salmon Garden Salad

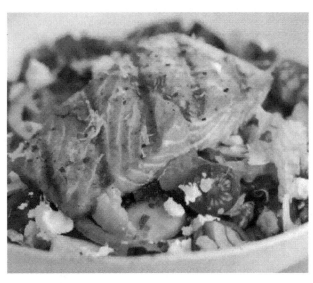

SERVES: 2
COOKING TIME: 10 MINUTES

INGREDIENTS:
- ½ pound salmon
- 1 cup of cucumber, peeled and diced
- 1 cup of diced fennel bulb
- 1 cup of diced red onions
- 2 tablespoons + 1 teaspoon olive oil, divided
- 3 tablespoons apple cider vinegar
- Pepper and salt to taste

METHOD
1. Preheat oven to 400oF. Grease a small baking dish with 1 teaspoon olive oil. Place salmon with skin side down and season with pepper and salt. Pop in preheated oven and bake for 8 to 10 minutes or until salmon is flaky.
2. Remove salmon from the oven. Coarsely flake salmon with two forks and discard skin of salmon. Let it cool.
3. Meanwhile, in a large salad bowl whisk well-remaining olive oil and vinegar. Toss in fennel, onions, cooled salmon, and cucumber. Toss to coat well and serve.

NUTRITION INFORMATION:
- Calories: per Serving: 362
- Carbohydrates: 18g
- Protein: 26g
- Fats: 21g
- Phosphorus: 396mg
- Potassium: 1157mg
- Sodium: 152mg

Kidney Disease Stage 3

51.   Rosemary Grilled Chicken

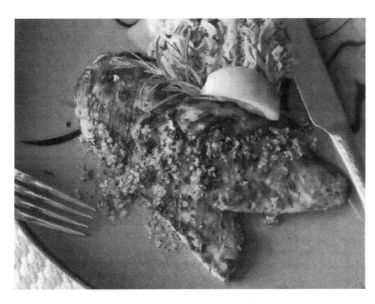

SERVES: 4
COOKING TIME: 12 MINUTES

INGREDIENTS:
- 1 tablespoon of fresh parsley, finely chopped
- 1 tablespoon of fresh rosemary, finely chopped
- 1 tablespoon of olive oil
- 4 pieces of 4-oz chicken breast, boneless and skinless
- 5 cloves of garlic, minced

METHOD
1. In a shallow and large bowl mix salt, parsley, rosemary, olive oil, and garlic. Place chicken breast and marinate in a bowl of herbs for at least an hour or more before grilling.
2. Grease grill grates and preheat grill to medium-high. Once hot, grill chicken for 4 to 5 minutes per side or until juices run a clear and internal temperature of chicken is 168oF.

NUTRITION INFORMATION:
- Calories: per Serving: 218
- Carbohydrates: 1g
- Protein: 34g
- Fats: 8g
- Phosphorus: 267mg
- Potassium: 440mg
- Sodium: 560mg

Kidney Disease Stage 5

52. Creamy Egg Scramble on Cauliflower Pilaf

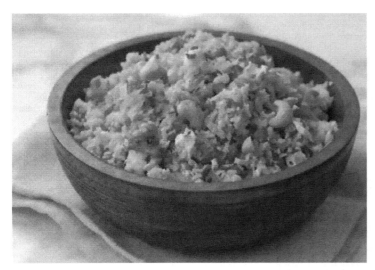

SERVES: 3
COOKING TIME: 25 MINUTES

INGREDIENTS:
- 1 head of cauliflower, trimmed and coarsely chopped
- 1 medium onion, diced
- 2 teaspoons of chives, chopped
- 3 tablespoons of olive oil, divided
- 4 eggs
- pepper to taste

METHOD
1. To make the cauliflower pilaf, place a nonstick large saucepan on medium fire and heat 2 tablespoons oil. Sauté onions until soft and translucent, around 10 minutes.
2. Meanwhile, process cauliflower in a food processor using the 'S' blade to create a bowl of rice textured cauliflower pilaf.
3. Add cauliflower pilaf to a pan of onions and cook until soft, around 5 to 10 minutes of sautéing. Season with pepper and mix well. Transfer pilaf and evenly divide into two dishes.
4. In the same pan, heat remaining oil on medium fire.
5. Whisk well eggs, pepper to taste and chives. Pour into heated oil and scramble for two or three minutes or to desired doneness. Once cooked, divide into two and top each plate of cauliflower pilaf with egg. Serve and enjoy.

NUTRITION INFORMATION:
- Calories: per Serving: 250
- Carbohydrates: 10g
- Protein: 10g
- Fats: 20g
- Phosphorus: 172mg
- Potassium: 447mg
- Sodium: 113mg

Kidney Disease Stage 4

53. Roasted Veggies Mediterranean Style

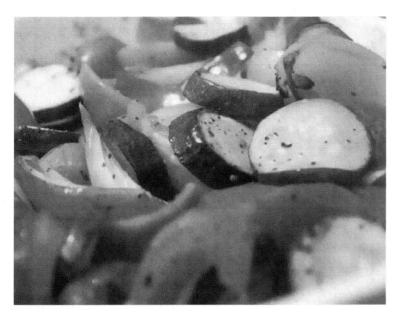

SERVES: 2
COOKING TIME: 10 MINUTES

INGREDIENTS:
- ½ teaspoon of freshly grated lemon zest
- 1 cup of grape tomatoes
- 1 tablespoon of extra-virgin olive oil
- 1 tablespoon of lemon juice
- 1 teaspoon of dried oregano
- 10 pitted black olives, sliced
- 12-oz of broccoli crowns, trimmed and cut into bite-sized pieces
- 2 cloves of garlic, minced
- 2 teaspoons of capers, rinsed

METHOD
1. Preheat oven to 350oF and grease a baking sheet with cooking spray.
2. In a large bowl toss together until thoroughly coated salt, garlic, oil, tomatoes, and broccoli. Spread broccoli on the prepped baking sheet and bake for 8 to 10 minutes.
3. In another large bowl mix capers, oregano, olives, lemon juice, and lemon zest. Mix in roasted vegetables and serve while still warm.

NUTRITION INFORMATION:
- Calories per Serving: 110
- Carbs: 16g
- Protein: 6g
- Fats: 4g
- Phosphorus: 138mg
- Potassium: 745mg
- Sodium: 214mg

Kidney Disease Stage 5

54. Fruity Garden Lettuce Salad

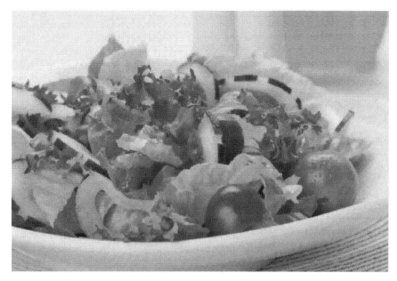

SERVES: 4
COOKING TIME: 0 MINUTES

INGREDIENTS:
- ¼ cup apple cider vinegar
- ¼ cup chopped almonds
- ½ avocado, thinly sliced
- ½ cup extra virgin olive oil
- ½ lemon, juiced
- 1 teaspoon ground black pepper
- 2 Granny Smith apples, thinly sliced
- 2 teaspoons grainy mustard
- 6 cups thinly sliced lettuce

METHOD
1. In a large salad bowl, toss lemon juice and apples. Mix in almonds, avocado, and lettuce.
2. In a small bowl mix salt, pepper, mustard, vinegar, and olive oil until salt is thoroughly dissolved.
3. Pour dressing over lettuce mixture and toss well to combine. Serve and enjoy.

NUTRITION INFORMATION:
- Calories per Serving: 123
- Carbs: 16.5g
- Protein: 2g
- Fats: 6g
- Phosphorus: 56mg
- Potassium: 450mg
- Sodium: 35mg

Kidney Disease Stage 1

55. Red Coleslaw with Apple

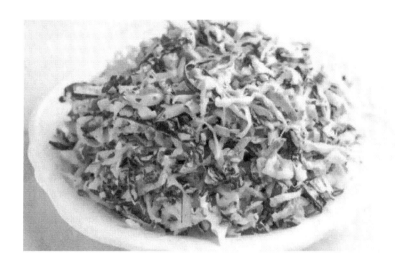

SERVES 4 • PREP TIME: 10 MINUTES

Loaded with anticarcinogenic, antibacterial, antiviral, and antioxidant properties, cabbage is a powerhouse vegetable and is terrific served raw. In this coleslaw, the red-cabbage variety (which is especially rich in antioxidants) pairs with a tart apple for a unique combination. Serve this salad alongside poultry, pork, or fish.

INGREDIENTS
- 3 cups of shredded red cabbage
- ½ cup of shredded carrots
- ¼ cup of finely chopped scallions
- Juice of 2 lemons
- 1 tablespoon of honey
- 1 tablespoon of extra-virgin olive oil
- 1 large tart apple, peeled and finely diced
- Freshly ground black pepper

METHOD
1. In a large bowl, add the cabbage, carrots, scallions, lemon juice, honey, olive oil, and apple. Mix well and refrigerate for 30 minutes to chill. Toss with black pepper right before serving.
2. Ingredient tip: Cabbage is sold in both red and green varieties. For this recipe, you will need less than a full head of cabbage, so if your store sells halved and wrapped cabbage, you can purchase this to avoid waste. Alternatively, you can save time by buying pre-shredded cabbage.

NUTRITIONAL INFO
- Per Serving Calories: 94
- Total Fat: 4g
- Saturated Fat: 1g
- Cholesterol: 0mg

- Carbohydrates: 16g
- Fiber: 3g
- Protein: 2g
- Phosphorus: 28mg
- Potassium: 303mg
- Sodium: 281mg

Kidney Disease Stage 1

56. Roasted Cauliflower with Mixed Greens Salad

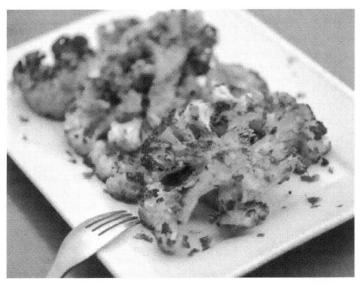

SERVES 4 • PREP TIME: 10 MINUTES
COOK TIME: 35 MINUTES

Mixed baby salad greens are ready for anything you throw at them. These mildly flavored greens shine in this simple salad, with just one other vegetable—cauliflower—competing for attention. Roasted until golden brown, the tender cauliflower florets are greeted with a light vinaigrette and a sprinkling of walnut pieces for added texture and protein in this lovely dinner accompaniment.

INGREDIENTS
- 1 small head of cauliflower, cut into small florets
- 2 tablespoons of extra-virgin olive oil, divided
- Freshly ground black pepper
- 6 ounces of mixed baby salad greens
- 2 tablespoons of walnut pieces
- 1 tablespoon of apple cider vinegar

METHOD
1. Preheat the oven to 400°F.
2. In a large bowl, toss the cauliflower with 1 tablespoon of olive oil. Season with pepper. Arrange in a single layer on a large baking sheet.
3. Cook for 30 to 35 minutes, stirring once or twice, until tender and golden brown. Let cool for about 10 minutes.
4. Meanwhile, in a small bowl, mix the remaining tablespoon of olive oil and the vinegar.
5. In a large bowl, toss the mixed salad greens, walnuts, and cauliflower. Just before serving, stir in the olive-oil-and-vinegar mixture, and season with pepper.
6. Cooking tip: Make some extra roasted cauliflower as a side, and keep some on hand to whip up this salad without the wait when you need it. It will keep in an airtight container in the refrigerator for three to five days.

NUTRITIONAL INFO
- Per Serving Calories: 108
- Total Fat: 9g
- Saturated Fat: 1g
- Cholesterol: 0mg
- Carbohydrates: 5g
- Fiber: 2g
- Protein: 2g
- Phosphorus: 42mg
- Potassium: 217mg
- Sodium: 50mg

Kidney Disease Stage 4

57. Bulgur and Broccoli Salad

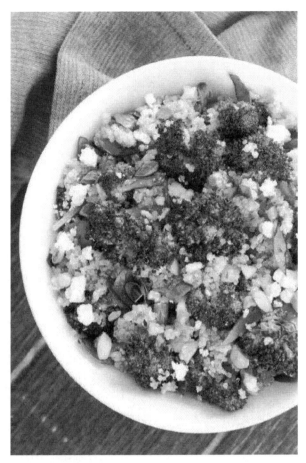

SERVES 4 • PREP TIME: 10 MINUTES
COOK TIME: 15 MINUTES

Mint may play a supporting role here, but this cooling herb adds immeasurable brightness to anything it touches. Here the mint is combined with lemon, broccoli, and cherry tomatoes to create a vibrantly flavored salad with the nutty-tasting bulgur at its base. Serve this salad on its own or spoon it into large lettuce leaves to create a tasty hands-on salad wrap.

INGREDIENTS

- 3 cups of broccoli florets
- 1 cup of bulgur
- ½ cup of cherry tomatoes halved
- ¼ cup of raw sunflower seeds
- ¼ cup of chopped mint leaves
- Juice of 1 lemon
- 1 tablespoon of extra-virgin olive oil

METHOD

1. In a medium bowl, prepare an ice-water bath by filling the bowl with ice and water.
2. Fill a medium pot halfway with water and bring to a boil. Add the broccoli and blanch for 3 minutes. With a slotted spoon, remove the broccoli and transfer it to the ice bath, retaining the cooking water over the heat. Once cool, after about 3 minutes, drain the ice and water. Set the broccoli aside.
3. Add the bulgur to the hot water, remove from the heat, cover, and let sit for 15 minutes. Drain, pressing the bulgur with the back of a spoon to remove excess moisture.
4. In a medium bowl, toss the broccoli, bulgur, tomatoes, sunflower seeds, mint, lemon juice, and olive oil. Serve immediately.

Ingredient tip: Bulgur can go rancid quickly, so buy only what you will use in the near future. If possible, smell it for freshness before purchasing, and store it in the refrigerator.

NUTRITIONAL INFO
- Per Serving Calories: 156
- Total Fat: 6g
- Saturated Fat: 1g
- Cholesterol: 0mg
- Carbohydrates: 24g
- Fiber: 7g
- Protein: 6g
- Phosphorus: 101mg
- Potassium: 315mg
- Sodium: 21mg

Kidney Disease Stage 1

58. Marinated Shrimp and Pasta

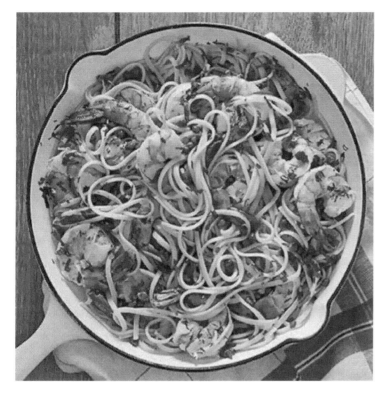

COOKING TIME: 10 MINUTES

DESCRIPTION

A hearty recipe that combines shrimps, pasta, and various veggies for a burst of colors and flavors. A great pasta salad dish for lunch and guest food.

INGREDIENTS FOR 10 SERVINGS

- 12 oz. of three-colored penne pasta
- ½ pound of cooked shrimp
- ½ red bell pepper, diced
- ½ cup of red onion, chopped
- 3 stalks of celery
- 12 baby carrots, cut into thick slices
- 1 cup of cauliflower, cut into small round pieces
- ¼ cup of honey
- ¼ cup of balsamic vinegar
- ½ tsp. of black pepper
- ½ tsp. garlic powder
- 1 tbsp. of French mustard
- ¾ cup of olive oil

METHOD

1. Cook pasta for around 10 minutes (or according to packaged instructions).
2. While pasta is boiling, cut all your veggies and place into a large mixing bowl. Add the cooked shrimp.
3. In a mixing bowl, add the honey, vinegar, black pepper, garlic powder, and mustard.
4. While you whisk, slowly incorporate the oil and stir well.
5. Add in the drained pasta with the veggies and shrimp and gently combine everything together.
6. Pour the liquid marinade over the pasta and veggies and toss to coat everything evenly.
7. Refrigerate for 3-5 hours prior to serving.
8. Serve chilled.

NUTRITIONAL INFORMATION (Per Serving)
- Calories: 256kcal
- Carbohydrate: 41g
- Protein: 6.55g
- Sodium: 242.04mg
- Potassium: 131.88mg
- Phosphorus: 86.03mg
- Dietary Fiber: 2.28g
- Fat: 16.88g

Kidney Disease Stage 3

59. Steak and Onion Sandwich

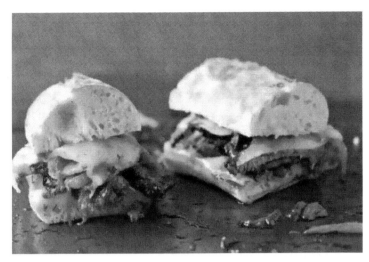

COOKING TIME: 8 MINUTES

DESCRIPTION

A rich steak sandwich that is very filling when you have to eat something good but don't have much time. Make this ahead for the next working day lunch or enjoy it fresh with the rest of your family.

INGREDIENTS FOR 4 SERVINGS

- 4 flank steaks (around 4 oz. each)
- 1 medium red onion, sliced
- 1 tbsp. of lemon juice
- 1 tbsp. of Italian seasoning
- 1 tsp. of black pepper
- 1 tbsp. of vegetable oil
- 4 sandwich/burger buns

METHOD

1. Wrap the steak with the lemon juice, the Italian seasoning to taste. Cut into 4 pieces
2. Heat the vegetable oil in a medium skillet over medium heat.
3. Cook steaks around 3 minutes on each side until you get a medium to well-done result. Take off and transfer onto a dish with absorbing paper.
4. In the same skillet, saute the onions until tender and transparent (around 3 minutes).
5. Cut the sandwich bun into half and place 1 piece of steak in each topped with the onions.
6. Serve or wrap with paper or foil and keep in the fridge for the next day.

NUTRITIONAL INFORMATION (Per Serving)

- Calories: 315.26 kcal
- Carbohydrate: 8.47 g
- Protein: 38.33 g
- Sodium: 266.24 mg
- Potassium: 238.2 mg
- Phosphorus: 364.25 mg
- Dietary Fiber: 0.76 g
- Fat: 13.22 g

Kidney Disease Stage 2

Shopping List

Vegetables
- Alfalfa sprouts Arugula
- Asparagus Bean sprouts
- Beets, canned
- Cabbage, green/red Carrots
- Cauliflower
- Celery
- Chiles
- Chives
- Coleslaw
- Corn
- Cucumber
- Eggplant
- Endive
- Ginger root
- Lettuce
- Onions
- Parsley
- Radishes
- Spaghetti squad
- Turnips
- Vegetables, mixed
- Water chestnuts, canned
- Bread and Cereals
- Cereals, Kellogg's
- Corn Flakes
- Cereals, Cheerios
- Cereals, Corn Chex

Beverages
- 7UP
- Coffee
- Cream soda
- Fruit punch
- Ginger ale

- Grape soda
- Hi-C
- Lemon-lime soda
- Lemonade
- Orange soda
- Root beer
- Tea

Dairy and Dairy Alternatives
- Almond milk
- Coffee-mate
- Mocha Mix
- Rice Dream
- Rich's Coffee Rich

Other
- Apple butter Corn syrup Honey
- Jam Jelly
- Maple syrup
- Sugar, brown or white sugar, powdered

TIME-SAVING STRATEGIES

If you are always on the go, with errands to run, dinner to make, and a schedule to maintain, grocery shopping can test your patience. Maintaining a healthy, appropriate diet comes down to effective meal planning and grocery shopping. While many people who don't have chronic kidney disease may buy food at random during the week, people with kidney disease need to do a bit more planning and have an effective grocery-store strategy.

Keep yourself on track with these six tips for efficient food shopping:

1. Don't shop on an empty stomach. Go shopping after you've eaten. This will help you avoid buying unhealthy food products.

2. Have your shopping list ready. Keep your grocery list organized and efficient, arranging items by category or grouping items that are usually found in the same aisle. There are two advantages to this trick: you spend less time in the grocery store, and you are less likely to forget something.

3. Plan ahead. Try to plan out your meals and foods for the week. It will save you time, and you won't stress out over daily menu planning.

4. Keep it simple. Your shopping trip doesn't have to be time-consuming. Do you have coffee, sugar, cereal, bread, fruit, or milk? What will you be packing for lunch? Do you have the recipe, so you can jot down the ingredients you need ahead of time?

5. Stick to the list. When you go to the grocery store, do not stray from your list. Avoid impulse buys because this will help you avoid unhealthy purchases and save you money.

6. Fresh is best. One of the best places to grocery shop is at your local farmers' market. Farmers' markets always have the freshest and most delicious produce. When you consider the value of organic, local foods, and their potential positive effect on your health, you won't mind paying a little more at the farmers' market.

Eating healthy and maintaining a diet that's kidney-friendly doesn't have to be hard. With the right amount of planning, a little prep work, and a good grocery-store strategy, creating a healthy meal plan can be easy and fun.

Made in the USA
Las Vegas, NV
16 September 2021